Resurrection of Health

A **NEW** Perspective for
Achieving & Mastering Your Wellness

Dr. Sian Comora

ISBN: 978-1-7370137-9-2

Mastering Wellness Publications
Sunland, California

Interior designed by Tami Boyce (tamiboyce.com)

This book is dedicated to my family:
Margaret, my dear mother;
my sweet father Emanuel;
my dearest and beautiful Sister's, Aileen and Madeleine;
and my charismatic, sweet, and funny nephews,
Kavi and Siva.

A **big Thank You** to Monty Cox, Cindy DeWeese Drake,
The Burkett Family, Nancy Zinner, and
everyone else who has been supportive to me along my journey.

Finally, a new perspective for mastering your wellness. A fun and delightful read woven with inspiration. Full of wisdom that will have a positive life-changing impact. Transmute, transform, and resurrect your health.

Margaret Comora
Mother
Musician/Teacher/Writer

This book is **NOT** intended for the treatment or prevention of disease, nor as a substitute for medical treatment, nor as an alternative to medical advice. It is for informational purposes only.

Table of Contents

Foreword

first met Sian Comora when running in the hills of Glendale, California. We have now been friends for quite some years. Not long after getting to know her, she shared with me her early life challenges with her health. It was one of those things where you say to yourself "was that really true? Could this be possible?" With a smile on her face and a 'child-like' fascination with life, one would never know the "story" of her life she carries with her. You can feel her renewed passion for living. She knows about living a life of sickness and now a life of wellness.

Upon getting to know her, I, being in an intense world of physicality my whole life, have learned so much from her. In a most joyful demeanor and in her simplistic and unique style of education, she started sharing her wealth of knowledge, knowledge which she shares in this book. She shared with me her biomedical research background at UCLA in Immunology and Clinical Oncology and her journey into the world of holistic medicine. *The coming together of these disciplines sets her apart.* While she is not against western medicine overall, her perspective from her experience is one to learn from. Common sense is woven into how the use of western/conventional and holistic practices can be used together to one's advantage.

Sian's experience is one that few practitioners can identify with. She can empathize first hand with the challenges people face to gain a better state of health—the confusion, frustrations, and wealth of mis-information. However, she can attest to the elation when goals are achieved. She can truly say *"she understands"* as she has lived on both sides of the fence, sickness and health. Her *compassion and empathy towards people is real*. When you meet her you immediately feel that.

Sian's story is real, heart-touching, and inspiring. Without even realizing it, your mind will be effortlessly trained to see health and wellness in a **new** way, a way that you will be able to apply, and which will remain with you for life, and change your life for the better. Honestly, without your health, you have nothing.

Monty Cox
2nd Unit Director
Stunt/Animal Coordinator
Stuntman
Former President, International
Stunt Association (ISA)

Foreword

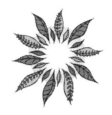

I met Dr. Sian before the 2012 summer Olympics. A colleague and friend of hers, an Elite, Olympic level coach in Track & Field and trainer, connected us. I was interested in receiving comprehensive information on alkaline, ionized water. Her knowledge in the various fields of molecular/cellular biology, biomedical research, and holistic health overall impressed me. After connecting with her over the phone, she arranged to visit me at the Olympic Training Center in Chula Vista. We arranged a full day visit to the center where I gave her a tour of the facilities and introduced her to athletes. She observed training on the track field and we sat and chatted at various times throughout the day on various topics from training to nutrition to psychology. I also got to hear her personal health story and journey to wellness at that time. Sian visited me and the athletes in Chula Vista at the training center many more times, came to watch track meets to support me and the athletes and we have since become very good friends.

Sian has written an excellent account of her personal health experience. Her life story expresses frustration, depression, financial hardship, wasted time, but in the end, elation. Had she found earlier in life what she found later in life as a cure, her life during those 20 years would have been so much richer and more rewarding in many ways.

This is a read for everyone. The reader will find her story fascinating and informative. It is packed with great educational knowledge anyone can relate to.

A found treasure for anyone who desires a fuller life.

Coach R. Craig Poole, Ed.D
Past Director/Head Coach Olympic Training Center, Chula Vista
Director of Sport Performance,
National Athletic Institute (NAI)
Elite Level III Track & Field Coach

Foreword

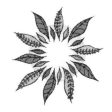

am Margaret Comora. I am 96 years old and have been a musician/teacher and writer. Sian is my youngest daughter of three. I am writing this foreword, not because she is my daughter, but because her health journey in her younger life has been an inspiration to me. I believe her story and advice will be fortifying, motivational, and inspirational for others as well. Those who know of it have told me this over the years.

Everyone has challenges and ups and downs throughout life, of course different for each and everyone of us and we experience them at varying times throughout our lives. We say everyone has a "story." I was a foster child given up by my own mother who never wanted me to know who my real birth father was. I channelled my hurt and pain into music - mainly the piano and cello. Even though I loved playing music I was attracted to teaching younger children the magic and beauty of music. I was also a writer. I had my own magazine column for years when I lived overseas. I lost my husband, and the children lost their father, 29 years ago. He suffered a massive heart attack in the middle of the day, no warning or notice. We had no idea he had left us until late that evening when a phone message was left on my answering machine asking me to come to the hospital and identify my husband in the morgue. What a heart-breaker to have to tell your children all of a sudden, their father is gone! Eight years ago, I lost my middle daughter, the girl's sister, to a rare illness picked up while traveling. She had twin boys who were only 5 years old at the time of her passing. How do you explain to six year old twins their mother has passed on.

Then there is the story of my youngest girl whose story you will read here. To see my youngest daughter suffer and experience childhood in a very differing way than what we would call 'normal,' was heart-wrenching, to say the least. It was a tumultuous path, struggling internally with my own voice questioning my actions as a parent. I witnessed and experienced alongside her father/my husband our child's pain, sorrow, sadness, and hurt. I never new at any point what the final outcome would be for my daughter. I never would have imagined her health would be restored as it was. What a colorful life I have lived thus far, experiencing the full gamut of situations and emotions from sorrow and pain to joy and amazement.

It has mesmerized me how we as humans, cope with such challenges throughout life. The word 'Resilience' comes to my mind. In most definitions it will say something like: "tending to recover from or adjust easily/quickly to misfortune or change." I would take out the words "easily and quickly." If referring to an object one usually sees the definition that says something like: "elasticity or the ability of a substance or object to spring back into shape." I think we can merge these definitions and associate them to how we cope as humans to trying situations. I have been resilient over the years, but so too have my children and grandchildren. We can, over time, re-shape ourselves, whether it be mental, physical, or emotional. Or using what my daughter writes about... *transmute and transform.* It is not an instant process, but just because it takes time —a different amount of time for each as an individual— doesn't mean it cannot happen.

I encourage you to read this book with an open mind and heart. I believe there is *wisdom* in it that will have a positive, life-changing impact.

Margaret Comora
Mother/Musician/Writer/Teacher

A Medical Prediction

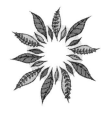

The final, definitive words spoken to me by a renowned MD specialist in his field who was treating me were:

"There is nothing more we can do for your chronic, life-threatening health condition. You are destined, in the very near future, to live in an indoor, air-purified bubble for the rest of your life, as you will NOT be able to breathe in the normal air around you."

I was 26 years young!

An Unusual Case

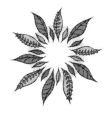

My chronic health challenges began when I was six years old. Because of breathing difficulties, I was unable to sleep in a normal, reclining position. My throat was sore and inflamed, my sinuses were extremely tender and blocked, my breathing was labored along with a heavy feeling in my chest, and I had tremendous pressure in my head. I could not sleep unless I was propped up with pillows, basically sleeping in an upright position.

From the time I woke up in the morning, the misery began. I would begin feeling allergic. I would start sneezing, my eyes would begin itching and watering, my sinuses were tender and began blocking up, my throat would begin swelling and becoming sore, and a major headache would ensue shortly after that, throbbing and pounding. I would also feel very lethargic. A short time after I got up and began my day, I felt as though a Mack truck had hit me. My head felt like a huge weight upon my shoulders; my whole body felt as though it were fighting a war.

My parents, very concerned about my health and how I was feeling, took me to the doctor. The doctor said I might have allergies and should see a specialist. My father, who was in the medical field (an oral surgeon), wanted to seek the best care for me and took me to an allergy specialist recommended to him by other top physicians. The specialist believed I indeed was suffering from allergies and recommended I be tested for allergies to a variety of pollens and foods.

The testing began with pollens and then proceeded to a number of foods that more commonly cause allergic responses. Several rows of scratch testing were done on the skin of my forearm with actual pollen from a long list of trees and grasses. The local allergic response, rated on a scale of 1 to 4, 4 being highly allergic, produced a circular, raised, red area almost like a big insect bite. The testing would begin at the top of the forearm just below the elbow, continue down to the wrist, and repeat several times, thus creating several rows of testing. Before they even reached the end of the first row of testing on the same arm, the areas were swelling to the top level of the 1-4 measuring scale. Since they could not fit all of the testing in with such a response, they would continue the testing on the other arm. In a very short period of time, I basically had numerous "welts" develop. Because I was so allergic, they then needed more room for the rest of the testing and went to my upper arms. When all the testing was done, the doctor would review the areas of my arms, scoring each spot from the 1 to 4-scale system, again 4 being highly allergic. About 95% of all the pollens tested on me scored a 3+ to 4.

Surprisingly, I was not allergic to any of the foods tested. The doctor was very surprised to see such strong allergic responses to so many pollens, especially at such a young age. I was an "unusual" case he stated; however, he assured me that I could be helped. He gave me some samples of anti-histamines to take right then in the office to counter my body's response to the testing. I was already beginning to feel the allergic affects of the testing, not only locally but systemically also.

The course of treatment he recommended was tri-weekly allergy shots of small amounts of these allergens (I would need several shots due to the fact that I was so allergic to such a large number of them). Daily antihistamines were recommended to manage additional symptoms. I was also given several cloth surgical masks. Yes, surgical masks! The doctor told my parents I should wear one when outdoors to help minimize exposure to the pollens during the initial period of treatment.

I began the recommended treatment that soon became a regular part of my life at this stage. Three times per week, my mother took me for my allergy shots. Antihistamines became a daily routine. When my sinuses or throat were inflamed, antibiotics were prescribed plus an assortment of over-the-counter remedies (e.g., nasal sprays, saline mists, etc.). Additional over-the-counter analgesics were recommended for my headaches at this time. If these did not alleviate my symptoms, a prescription would be given.

Months and months went by. I thought I was improving somewhat, but I was still suffering from the same symptoms I originally developed. At times I felt worse over all. Without realizing it, I was trying to convince myself it wasn't so bad. I was becoming accustomed to the symptoms that constantly plagued me--I was becoming uncomfortably comfortable. I continued to be extremely fatigued throughout the day which lead to the need to take an extended nap in the afternoon. I barely made it home from my school day before my body went into an exhaustive, shutdown mode.

Every few months, back to the doctor I went. Every few months I was also re-tested to check for improvements, but only a few tested pollens seemed to improve slightly. The doctor's recommendations again were to continue the shots and antihistamines. Again, antibiotics were prescribed when my throat and sinus problems arose. His advice was, "Be patient. You are a **very unusual case**," reassuring me and my parents that everything was working well.

Months turned into several years. Every few months I returned to the doctor for re-testing. At this point they began adding a few more pollens that were prevalent for the season and which they thought might additionally pose a problem. Sure enough, I was very allergic to these. Along with this, I showed only a minute improvement in my tested response to a few pollens. I was still in misery following the testing. The pollens tested were still scoring a 3+ to 4 and now they needed my whole upper back area for testing because of the vigorous response. I needed to take an even higher dose of antihistamines to counter the allergic response to the testing. I also had to remain in the doctor's office to be observed, to make sure I was alright. In spite of the fact that these tests revealed no significant improvement and my symptoms were not clearing up (they were basically barely being managed, if that), the doctor's recommendations were again the same: "continue the shots and antihistamines, be patient and he repeated in amusement, you are a **very unusual case.**" There was, however, a new magical statement of "so far this year we are experiencing an especially bad allergy season. The pollen counts are unusually higher this year." He recommended that my father have some vials of epinephrine for injection on hand at home just in case I had an "unusually" severe systemic allergic reaction one day. He extended his recommendations even further and suggested my father teach me how to inject myself with the epinephrine. He also advised that I carry a vial and syringes with me and make sure my school was aware of my condition. He still recommended I wear the surgical mask, directing that it *must* be put on prior to going outside, and to continue wearing it to minimize the amount of pollens inhaled outdoors. Despite all this, he still commented that I was doing extremely well! This was improvement! Looking back now, this was the *insanity* that was developing with my health-care treatment.

As time went on, my symptoms were escalating, older ones intensifying and new ones appearing. There were days when I just could not bear to go outside. I would feel so miserable that I would try to avoid it. The surgical masks became a regular wardrobe accessory. There were also days that I definitely could not go outdoors as I was so allergic that my body could not tolerate the air—it was not safe for me. There was considerable concern that even though I knew how to inject myself with epinephrine, if I were on my own, I might not be able to do so in a timely manner. I was living in **terror** of what the air would be like outside. Over the years, not only was the time I could spend outdoors nonexistent or significantly reduced, but my enjoyment of playing outdoors, if I could, became a burden of fear. I felt I was being robbed of precious childhood fun. All the while I kept convincing myself that I was feeling a bit better, possibly a false sense of security that I was creating to override the fears that were developing .

On a daily basis I was now petrified with this fear of what the air outside was like and whether my body could handle breathing it. The allergic response by my body was extremely intense and I had no control over it. My life was in danger once I ventured outside. My body's reactions were not only more intense, but they were coming on more quickly upon my exposure to the air. Now, within seconds of going outside, an allergic response developed. I would begin sneezing profusely and my face would begin swelling, my eyes would also begin swelling and puffing up, and itching, burning, and watering would follow. My breathing became sluggish; sometimes I felt like I was being suffocated. I became so scared that I was almost in complete panic. The headaches were more intense and lasting longer. Throbbing sharp pains would radiate up and across my sinuses along with extreme tenderness. Every day my ear canals were now becoming blocked, I had constant pressure, my throat was always red, sore, and inflamed and I was constantly clearing mucous from it. If that weren't enough, I was now getting intensified throat infections with huge, painful ulcers on my tonsils. (On a side note, I still had my tonsils and it was advised that they remain because as part of the immune system, they provide some filtering protection). Breathing had become extremely labored and wheezy. In addition, I had developed a chronic cough, one that caused other children in school to move away from me in class.

My antihistamine dose needed to be increased, but with caution because there were times when my heart would flutter. My father discussed with the doctor if this were really safe; his response was, "Well, we will see, but she should try not to take the higher dose too often." Again, looking back, this was the continued insanity diffused through the "care" I was receiving. In general, the antihistamines contributed to *severe* dehydration (e.g. leg cramps) and made me tired on top of the extreme fatigue I had from the allergies. I was really getting minimal relief from them; yet, I had great fears about reducing them or not taking them at all. Great! Now, added fears complicated the situation even further. Should I even take the medication which supposedly would help my condition, but which makes me feel worse over all? If I don't take it, would it be risky? If I do take it, is it risky? Isn't this interesting? Constant dialogue was going on in my head over this, exhausting me even further. Antibiotic courses prescribed for my throat and sinuses became longer. At this point, I was really not getting much relief from all the allergy shots either. Fortunately, as I mentioned, my father taught me how to give myself an epinephrine shot in the event of an allergic emergency—I still carried it with me along with a small syringe everywhere I went (they did not have the epinephrine single dose injection pen at that time). People who knew me were aware of this also in case I needed assistance from them. Daily I prayed I would be okay and not need it. If I did need it, I prayed for the narrow window of time to administer it and get it into my system.

At this stage, my father was alarmed because I was only 14 years old and while my treatment initially helped to a degree, I had now come to a plateau and was heading downhill rapidly. The treatment plan was not working. He and my mother were heartbroken to see me suffer as I did. My father arranged an appointment with my allergy specialist to review my case with him. To his absolute amazement and sheer shock, so to speak, the doctor's advice was that we probably should re-test. With stern confidence, he insisted that the treatment was working, but we needed to be patient. My father commented that it had been eight years, I was suffering tremendously, and I was worse at this point. This was not at all congruent with the doctor's so-called treatment plan and expected outcome that was boasted about to us originally and over the years. Again, the doctor repeated, "Your daughter's case is an **unusual one**." She is the most allergic patient I have ever seen in my practice so far. The magical statement again surfaced: "The allergy season this year has been an *especially* bad one, posing a lot of trouble for people like your daughter who are highly allergic." My father remarked that this is what he had said every year when he had questioned my progress. The doctor never extended himself beyond this statement to even question what else might possibly be done for me. My father was now questioning his competence. My father was emphatic that we needed a better solution and he would find it. At this point he felt that this doctor was not at all concerned about my health. Instead of taking a more active role he was distancing himself and had become nonchalant. Defensive, offended, and cold would also be descriptive of his demeanor now. It seemed that I was now a number, not a person.

One Week At a Time

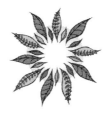

Back to the drawing board my father went. He began doing research on my health challenges, collecting names of new doctors, and making inquiry calls to other health practitioners he knew in hopes of finding a new physician and a better solution. During this time, another health challenge of mine that had been gaining momentum was now overwhelming. Over the years, blocked sinuses and ear pressure were constant symptoms. Now, the pressure had intensified to a point where it was painful and it was affecting my hearing. While my father was engaged in his research, one of the doctors he had known from New York, whom he was consulting with, recommended he take me to a prominent, well-known hearing institute in Los Angeles. An appointment was made and off we went when the time came. What a day this was! Just after arriving and signing in, off they took me, on my own. I was taken to one room after another where test after test was performed by a technician. Hour after hour went by while no one even explained what was going on. I had not even seen a doctor yet either. Eventually, they reunited me with my father and after an extended waiting period we were called into the doctor's office. Without any formal introduction on his part, just an abrupt "hello," nor a discussion of how I was feeling or case history questions, he fired off the diagnosis. In a matter of fact tone, he told us that I was losing my hearing. We were told that in a matter of months deafness would ensue. He handed my father and me literature regarding the onset of deafness and mentioned the need for our preparation for the inevitable result. My father tried to inform him of my serious allergic condition, which was also on the medical history we filled out, and inquired whether or not any of that had been looked at or evaluated by him. The doctor rapidly dismissed any allergy connection whatsoever and made no further attempt to discuss the situation. He was basically finished with our "brief" consult and out the door he went. My father was absolutely outraged, to say the least. We immediately left and as we did, I kept asking my father why the doctor did not even inquire about how I had been feeling before experiencing these symptoms or discuss my present state of health at all. Wow, I thought; this is what you call a prestigious institute? Throughout the whole drive home my father was trying, in any way he could, to comfort me. He said "this is only one opinion, and even though they have a supposedly good reputation, this does not mean they can't be incorrect." A constant stream of tears was running down my cheeks; I was in complete disbelief as to what was going on with my health. When we arrived home and shared this information with my mother, she said she felt skeptical about the results. She encouraged and urged my father to continue seeking new specialists in the allergy and immunology fields. My father did and he finally came across an allergy and immunology specialist who had a commendable reputation for more advanced, challenging cases. He arranged for us to see him.

Upon our first visit, the doctor himself was quite surprised to see the extent of my medical file. He wanted to review, more thoroughly, all the allergy testing and results in my file. After reviewing my file, he agreed that my case was very, very unusual. In spite of this, he began to inform us that there had been advancements in treatment on several fronts. The type of serums they were making for injections and the treatment protocols had improved. Also, there were newer medications and nasal inhaler sprays which blocked more specific responses in the cascade of reactions involved in the allergic response, thus helping to manage symptoms more effectively. He wanted to do some additional testing, but for only a select few components that he suspected might be giving me problems. For example, dust mites which are considered an environmental allergen. The other components were several common bacteria that are naturally found in the air and are benign for healthy people. This was a shocker to us. Dust mites, okay, but I might be allergic to common bacteria in the air? Goodness, the air I breathed was truly my enemy! He said that if this were the case, we would have a good handle on how to proceed. We were optimistic and chose to have him take over my case. When we additionally related the recent report from the hearing institute, he immediately examined my ears. His pronouncement was (almost laughing) that of course I could not hear because my ear canals were inflamed, swollen and totally blocked from the allergies. He attributed the institute's findings to incompetence and predicted that the hearing would normalize once the allergies were under control. Down the road, under his treatment protocol this proved to be true for the most part; however, although I continued to have constant ear pressure and swelling, my hearing was not impaired as before.

Well, wouldn't you know it? The new test results were amusing to say the least. Low and behold, I was also reacting to additional substances! My portfolio of allergens just got even bigger. Neither my father nor I thought it could possibly extend further. I was literally allergic to my environment—common bacteria found in the air. I had no normal immunity to four kinds of common bacteria. I couldn't escape this. The doctor informed us that this was causing the more intense symptoms (including the chronic cough plus the secondary throat/sinus infections) and why I was not improving as expected. He also informed us that Stanford Medical Center was the only place he was aware of on the West Coast that could prepare a special serum for the common airborne bacteria. It would be costly, though, several thousand dollars for just a few vials. The doctor felt I would really benefit and gain relief and recommended we try it for at least six months. We were all in agreement. At this point my parents, as well as I, were willing to try anything new.

Upon arrival of the new serums, my treatment plan was to receive these shots plus the other antigens (all the pollens) weekly. As I built up my resistance over a period of time, the shots would slowly be decreased and I would receive a maintenance shot every month or few months depending on how I was doing. Eventually, the goal was to be able to stop all the shots once my body had developed a substantial resistance. I was thrilled to hear this, but with underlying skepticism at the same time. Did I really believe that I could improve? No shots at all down the road? My belief system was divided, with excitement on one hand and gloomy hopelessness on the other.

Treatment began, and there I was again in the doctor's office every week. My father would say to me, "Take it one week at a time," and I would repeat that to myself over and over again. I was still in need of antihistamines that were prescribed for me, newer versions that were supposed to be more effective and hopefully did not cause heart flutters. New nasal sprays were also prescribed to control symptoms. They seemed to help a bit, but the "effects" (so-called side effects) on my body were heavy duty. My body did not like these at all. I began swelling up and getting bloated. I started gaining weight from them and I experienced great fatigue. My breathing became more labored, my whole body was constantly stiff and aching, and my muscles were cramping. The effects of these medications were worse than the relief they were supposed to bring. My father was concerned, consulted with the doctor and asked that I not be prescribed these. If the new shots began to work as they should, then it was reasonable to assume that I could manage without these inhalers. The doctor agreed but with a precautionary lecture and hesitation. Any throat or sinus infections along the way would still be dealt with by taking prescribed antibiotics. This was the same routine as previous years.

Over a few months, to my absolute surprise, I gradually began improving. My symptoms were still present, however, but they were diminishing in severity just slightly. The improvement was slow but steady. My resistance built up over several years and the doctor then began reducing the shots. As time progressed I eventually reached that "maintenance" phase I thought was so elusive. I was elated. I kept wondering if this was really true or whether I was dreaming. This was an absolute delight for me. Excitement and hope emerged, taking over the initial deeply engrained feelings of hopelessness. For the first time since having these health challenges, my life routine did not revolve around receiving injections. More importantly, I slowly became more confident in breathing the air around me. Imagine that! ***Having to acquire*** *confidence in breathing the air around me.* I actually felt a bit more "normal." I was still taking antihistamines and over-the-counter analgesics, but in reduced doses, and occasionally I did still get throat and sinus infections which were treated with antibiotics. These were milder compared to the previous years of agony and suffering.

I continued to feel pretty good over all and my condition was being managed quite well. My allergy conditions were finally under control.

The Merry-Go-Round of Insanity

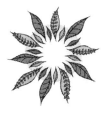

Years passed and then, at the height of my excitement about feeling good, things began shifting in an unusual way.

All kinds of new health challenges began popping up. I started getting intense, chronic yeast infections. They would be treated, go away, and then several weeks later they would return, more intense and lasting for a longer duration. Bladder infections started. I would get treated for those, they would stop, and then several weeks later they would return, more intense and for a longer duration. Headaches returned but they were not the same as they had been previously. These were even more intense, with sharp and throbbing pains that were now constant all day long. My ear canals began blocking up again, but I was now experiencing ringing in my ears. As if that were not enough, the severe dehydration escalated. In spite of drinking water by the gallons, my mouth and throat were so dry that I could barely pry my mouth open to talk, and my body literally felt like a fish drying up out of water.

Continuous, intense muscle cramping ensued as well (from my toes all the way up through my leg to my hips!). The dehydration interfered with my sleep, awakening me on a regular basis, thus compounding my over all exhaustion. I had big pitchers of water at my bedside at night in hope that it would relieve the symptoms. I even began developing numerous cavities in my teeth and ulcers in my mouth that were ascribed to the severe dehydration. Slowly, the throat infections began creeping back into the picture. I was treated with more antibiotics; the infections would resolve, but then return with a vengeance. At this point in time, I didn't realize that all the antibiotic treatments were contributing to many of these problems (e.g. chronic yeast and bladder infections). The prolonged use of antihistamines contributed to chronic dehydration issues and who knows what other health challenges. Additionally, a host of digestive problems had been developing along the way as well.

At this point I felt like I was on a merry-go-round with these new health challenges, spinning around faster and faster, and I could not get off the ride! Up the horse went, then down the horse went; around and around the merry-go-round went. I barely had one of these new health challenges under control when another one would pop up. One would go away and then another would pop up. I was given medication after medication to control one challenge and then the other and so on. Round and round, up and down, health challenge after health challenge, again and again. On and on it went.

I was extremely frightened! Major exhaustion from sickness was consuming me and I was downright depressed. It was at this point I began to really question what my body was going to do. Could it support all these challenges or would it be overwhelmed and completely shut down? Added to my emotional and physical

state at this point was severe anxiety about how I could continue to handle all this and cope with how I was feeling. My father
would say, "Let's take it one day at a time. We will find a solution."
Bless my father for his relentless support!

That's what I did. I took it one day at a time until things shifted again.

Insanity Still Prevailing

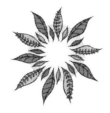

thought I had reached rock bottom. Then, to my absolute amazement, after pondering how anything else could happen, it did. I slowly became allergic to my surroundings again. My allergy symptoms and suffering began returning slowly but steadily. However, as the symptoms returned this time, they again seemed to be even more intense over all. As mentioned above, it was a pattern I had been experiencing continuously.

So back to the specialist we went. He was surprised, to say the least, but assured us that he could get me back to feeling better. This was just a little lapse and there was nothing to worry about. A little lapse? Nothing to worry about? My internal thoughts were, "It's not your body; I know how I have been feeling and this is not *little!*" Now I stepped forth and questioned him as to why I was plagued with all of these additional health challenges mentioned above and whether that related to the actual treatments for my allergies. I also questioned him about why the treatment plan he recommended worked for a period of time but then stopped. I mentioned that maybe all the treatment was overkill. Maybe I was getting too many shots over the years, adversely affecting my health and actually suppressing my system. His response was an emphatic "no." His voice was cool and calm about this and he had a smirky smile. His comments felt condescending, as though he were laughing at my inquiries. A bit like "How would she know? She is not a doctor." "We just need to retest you," he said, "start you back on new serums and frequent injections again for a bit, and get you onto a whole new arsenal of medications. They have developed much more effective medications over the past few years: the first non-drowsy antihistamine to new inhalers that block a different avenue of the allergic response cascade pathway." **Nothing to worry about** was my specialist's motto. I had heard this before. In my mind I said to myself, "Is he actually listening to what he is saying?" There was nothing new here and I was feeling like, "Oh no, here we go again." I repeatedly questioned him again as to why I had all these other health problems in addition to the allergies. This went right over him as though I had never asked a thing. That smile on his face was still there. I did not get any answers. I did not know what to do nor did my father at this point (although he did not let me know this), and so I went through the new testing. Yes, the insanity was still prevailing.

So there I was, back on a hefty treatment plan for the allergies, in addition to all the other infections and challenges mentioned above. Month after month I struggled. My father's health insurance company began writing letters to him that my specialist was charging too much for the medical treatments (at that time my medical expenses were thousands of dollars per month over the allowed coverage). My doctor would write letters back in support of the charges with copies of my medical file attached, saying "In all my professional years, I have never seen a patient like this. This patient should be in every medical textbook; she is an extremely unique case." She happens to be allergic to the majority of her surroundings; no normal person is like this, thus why the treatment is costing so much."

So how was I feeling now? **Absolutely horrible.** My condition was hardly being managed this time around. I don't think 'managed' even describes the situation at all. The enemy, my environment, was taking over the battle; I was losing the battle. Again there were days at a time, sometimes weeks or more, where venturing outside was risky for my health; I had to remain indoors. The surgical mask, my personal wardrobe accessory, was not even helping. My battle, though, was indoors too as the air I was breathing was also my enemy. So what could I do now?

My Enemy,
The Environment

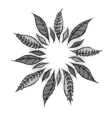

I was receiving all this treatment from top doctors and yet my condition continued getting worse. None of this made sense to me or to my father. What do we do; where do we turn at this point? My father was so determined to help me that again he went on a search for another doctor. Looking back now, this was the most familiar action to take. You just keep plodding along, knowing things are not quite right and not satisfied with the outcome but you stay on the same path. So, searching my father went; I followed along.

He found another highly recommended physician and off we went. My father was reassuring, but I was so miserable. I was virtually numb emotionally at this point. The physician was so eager to review my case for its "uniqueness" that he could not wait to jump right in. Jump in he did, enthusiastically. His recommendation was that I needed a different series of shots and regimen, the most up-dated in the field of allergy and immunology. This field has come a long way with more effective serums plus newer medications which are much more effective. They do not make you drowsy and the effects last for a longer period of time. Wow! Am I really hearing this or am I crazy? Have I heard this routine before? Or was I missing something and this was a new spiel on an old theme? Oh well, three is a charm, so this must be it this time, right? Just go along with it.

My father's recommendation was to try it. What else were we going to do? See what happens with the testing and his suggested protocol. I consented and treatment began. At first, I got frequent shots in the office. They were special serums again. I needed to be monitored very closely because of my severe condition so they kept me in the office for some time after administering the shots. The plan was again to build my resistance with this newer technique and then followup with less frequent maintenance shots. This was the new twist by this specialist? Had I heard this before or again, maybe I did not hear quite right? Of course, I also needed to take the "new" antihistamines on the market. Why? To manage all that was not covered by the shots—brilliant I thought!

So how did I feel after time on this course? —pretty much the same as before. I had become quite good at this point convincing myself I felt great. As time went on, it was apparent I was not improving. The doctor and his staff could see I was completely wiped out from not feeling well and that I was dragging myself through the office on the verge of collapsing. The travel time to this office for my treatment was a considerable distance also. It was all taking a toll on my body. The doctor said he was concerned about this and he recommended that because I was so knowledgeable about what was going on and had given myself injections before, he would let me take the serums home and do the injections myself. This took me by surprise. I asked him if that was safe. I thought this very odd because as I mentioned, they would not even let me leave the office for a considerable time after they injected me. Now he was saying that it was okay for me to inject myself at home? I began feeling as though he really had no time for any of this and no idea what to do; and so he thought, "let's just send her away." If she is not all right, she just won't be back. Yeah, right, I'll be in the hospital if I survive at all! He did not like my asking any questions about either this or my treatment in general, just like the other doctors. Now he was coming across as smug and arrogant, possessing the same attitude as the other doctor: mainly, what could I know; I'm not a doctor. I was given a host of instructions with precautions and warnings all over again. They went over the risks and signs of what I should do in case of an emergency. I kept asking them how this was even safe. "No worries," the office said, "You will just need to be stocked with epinephrine!" Off they sent me with a bag filled with serums, epinephrine, and syringes. The whole way home I kept thinking, "Are they just trying to kill me?" Of course not, I will be okay; they said I would. But then I would say to myself, "Wait a minute; you were not allowed to leave the office after your shots and now they are sending you home to administer the shots yourself." Back and forth my mind went, trying to reason and sort out what this was all about. Without resolution I arrived at home. Straight to the refrigerator I went and put the "goodies" inside. (I was trying to live a bit more on my own then, in our guesthouse just across the yard). I explained everything to my father that night and he was stunned also. The very next day I was scheduled to have my shots. I was petrified to inject myself and said again to myself out loud, "Can this be safe?" I waited for an answer from a higher intelligence. I did not get a good, comfortable feeling about doing this at all so I told my father he needed to be there. He adamantly agreed. He did not like the idea of home injections and said he should always be present. He was **always** there for me. After I gave myself the shots he sat with me for almost an hour. I now mentioned to my father that I was so angry and thoroughly disgusted with the whole situation. I felt none of these doctors were listening to me and they seemed not to care at all. I felt hopeless, lifeless, and told my father that if I did the injections, had a severe reaction and didn't come through, maybe that would be better as it would end all of this. I was, understandably, emotionally spent and confused. Over the years I trembled with such fear every day that it completely paralyzed me. This was accompanied by waves of sheer numbness, leaving me in a zombie-like state. All these precious, young years of my life I was barely getting through each day. I was completely zoned out from not feeling well, my body was breaking down from all the years on medications, and I was basically in a stupor. Everything seemed like a monumental effort. I was so tired of being sick and tired. Oddly enough, there was a part of me that continued trying to convince myself I felt okay! I was feeding this line so much to my subconscious over and over throughout the years that I wonder if this was a contributing factor as to why I never followed a different path for resolving my health challenges. The brilliant subconscious can stand ground, doing its highest work like a con artist, making you believe something is wonderful and great but that is just not true. This keeps one in a state of being uncomfortably comfortable. My father was upset also and very displeased with the doctors' attitudes and the profession at large. However, he never personally showed this to me during those years as he did not want me to ever get discouraged.

Things were not looking up in a very short period of time while seeing this doctor. My health was progressing even more rapidly in the opposite direction. I mustered all of my energy and went back to the doctor with my father, allergic to the environmental world around me and with a layering of intense health challenges all discussed previously. Oh yes, what a pleasant surprise when a new health problem arose. I was now having kidney problems! I looked like death warmed over; I was almost unrecognizable. I was not even sure I could make it to the doctor! I prayed for a speck of light and energy to keep me going for a bit longer. Just get me to the doctor. I felt worse than I ever had. To the doctor I posed questions again and again regarding my condition and my treatment. Why were all these other health challenges arising in addition to the allergies? Why would I improve a bit and then plateau? Maybe my system was getting over-stimulated or suppressed with all the shots? Maybe I am being over-medicated? How do you know this is not the case? To all of this, the answers by the doctor were, "We (medicine collectively) know what we are doing." "We just have to keep up the treatment." What "treatment?" That was my question. I am not being treated, for treatment means that improvement ensues. I am not improving. Not only am I not improving from the original health challenges, but the host of other health problems, never present originally, that had developed were not being "treated" either. I said to the doctor, "You are not even acknowledging those, let alone treating them. I have to keep pestering you to even listen." I was furious now; so, too, was my father. I now felt that since the first visit with this specialist, he was so enthusiastic about my "unusual case" not because he felt he could actually help me, but because he saw dollar signs all over the case. My father was in agreement about this. He did not even come close to his "reputation" and, in fact, helped me less than the previous specialist. He again just smiled and said, "Let me have the nurse check on your injection schedule and medications." He left the room. I started crying profusely. If this wasn't bad enough, when the nurse walked in, she did not even mention the schedule or my medications but instead asked, "are we scheduling another appointment for you?" She sounded like a recorded message, as if no human were even present. I looked straight at her with tears in my eyes as we passed her and just left the room. I wanted to say to her, "Is this a joke?" We walked passed the front desk and the office assistant there asked the same thing, "When are we seeing you again?" We still did not answer and walked out of the office. I completely broke down once outside. How did my father react? He tried to reassure me with, "don't lose hope, sweet pea."

Not long after this last appointment and all my questioning, my father received a phone call from the doctor directly. He asked to schedule an appointment with both of us present. My father made the appointment and we followed through.

That was the day. The doctor sat us down in his office and said:

> "There is nothing more we can do for your chronic, life-threatening health condition. You are destined, in the very near future, to live in an indoor, air-purified bubble for the rest of your life, as you will **NOT** be able to breathe in the normal air around you. I suggest you begin preparing your-self now."

I was absolutely shocked. Of course I felt as though the whole spirited essence of life had left my body in an instant. I began crying hysterically. My father was speechless. I could tell he was furious at the doctor. He said to him, "It seems like you really mis-led us from the start. Were you aware that your treatment options would not help?" My father felt there really was nothing more to say to the doctor. We walked out of the office. The whole time my father was trying to calm me down and he held his arms around me as though he were an angel carrying me under his wings. He said, "Let's go across the street for a bite to eat and sit and talk." While sitting in the restaurant, my father said to me with a big smile on his face while tears gushed down my face, "Don't worry; we **will** find help for you. Remember, don't give up hope."

Where Did the Angel Go?

About a week later, my angel left. My father passed away suddenly from a massive heart attack in the middle of the day. Neither I nor my family had any idea what had happened to him until that evening. My angel was just beginning to embark on another journey with me to find a new health solution. I was absolutely terrified, for my closest advocate on my behalf was no longer immediately by my side. Suddenly, my angel departed. Could I possibly now fly on my own?

I was shocked and in complete disbelief over my father's sudden passing. It was amazing, though, that I automatically went into survival mode for a short time. A few days after his passing, I was out of my antihistamines. Completely unable to think clearly about what to do, I just followed the path of least resistance and continued doing what I had been doing. I went to the pharmacy to pick up my prescription. It was the most recent antihistamine on the market, the first of its kind, what was called 'non-drowsy.' I had been taking this for several months since it came out on the market. I really did not feel a difference, but still plodded along the same path, regularly popping the pills. While waiting in the pharmacy for the prescription to be filled, I looked at the receipt and the slip of paper provided with the medication showing the so-called "side effects." The list was long, in fact, longer than I had remembered when it was previously filled. I had never really paid any close attention to the list, but just passed my eyes over it in one glance. This time I actually read through the list; I was checking off in my mind how many of these effects were exactly what I was experiencing. It was pretty much every one! Then I noticed one of the new side effects listed were kidney problems. That was it! I felt nauseous and my mouth dropped open, for I had been experiencing these problems and had kept asking the doctor about it. Never once had he even mentioned my kidney problems might be related to the side effects of the medication I was taking, perhaps not a "side effect" as is written or talked about, but the "effect" the medication has on the body. Because of my emotional state, I was barely able to process this; without realizing it, I was making note of all this subconsciously.

That night I cried myself to sleep. When I awakened the next morning, all I could do was just lie there. Deep, dark gloom and despair had set in. I had not even one ounce of desire to get up out of bed. I felt life was not worth living. I was having a breakdown. I was in shock and felt emotionally broken, not only over my father's passing, of course, but also over the doctor's words the previous week and over how I felt in general. I could not stop repeating in my mind, over and over, what the doctor had said about my condition: "you will be living inside an air-purified bubble for the rest of your life." I also kept asking why my father, my angel, flew away. At that moment all was hopeless. I felt there was nowhere to turn. I was shaking, and I still could not stop the deluge of tears flowing from me.

I tried to keep forcing myself to close my eyes and picture my father right in front of me with that smile on his face saying, "Don't worry; we will find you help. Don't give up hope." I prayed for help and relief. What do I do, angel who left me, what do I do? I kept repeating, "What do I do? " A statement from one of my favorite authors then suddenly popped into my head and I adopted it as my mantra. I recited it over and over again. This beautiful statement was:

**"Thou in me art divine inspiration,
revelation, and illumination."**

Over and over again I kept reciting it, asking the universe for guidance and what to do. I also kept asking my "angel," my father. Later that day, while still reciting my mantra the word "BALANCE" came to my mind. Balance related to my body. I then asked myself, "What about balance?" I continued to stay focused on my mantra and then came the words of "DAILY BALANCE." The body is striving for balance, Homeostasis, on a daily basis. I suddenly realized it was an absolute miracle that I was still even alive, let alone functioning at all. In spite of all the suffering I had endured and was enduring, my body had not given up on me. Despite challenge after challenge, year after year, even with all the allergy shots administered (who knows what other substances were in the vials in addition to the antigens) and copious amounts of toxic drugs put into my body, it had endured and kept trying to establish Homeostasis. All the symptoms were the expression of my body's attempts to stay balanced, shifting and re-shifting physiologically, treatment after treatment. It kept trying to regain that Homeostasis which is vital to life, no matter what the cost. My body, the human body, is absolutely amazing! It tries, in whatever manner it can, to keep its Homeostasis-balance. Regardless of how we feel, it is striving to maintain this for our existence every second throughout the day.

Now what? At this time it occurred to me that in the last year I had known something was seriously off with my treatments, either subconsciously or intuitively; this was the reason I kept questioning the doctor about over-medicating and possibly over-stimulating or suppressing my body's functioning with all the injections and drugs. How was it that initially I had allergies to environmental pollens, but that sphere of allergies kept expanding to more and more pollens, other environmental agents, and bacteria in the air that are normally benign to the body? Alongside of this was the development and expansion of all types of health challenges that were completely unrelated to the allergies. The doctors had NO explanation for this! No common sense knowledge ever even permeated their thinking with regard to all the drugs prescribed and their side-effects. Had they never, ever, read any of the descriptive information or warnings about the prescribed drugs' effects? They have big, fat Physician Desk Reference books in their office (PDR). I guess they never learned how to use those; maybe they do not even know what they are! And yes, they did not read any information about the drugs given to them at the time they received copious amounts of samples from the drug companies. They were, for the most part, too busy to be bothered and relied upon an overly abbreviated statement from either the company or a representative. In all likelihood, they just turned their heads away. Remember also that the doctors didn't even want to acknowledge the existence of any of these other health challenges. They would not even venture to investigate or question their procedures to figure out why I was becoming more and more allergic and being plagued with the plethora of additional health problems. I thought it was their job. We seek their services to help us. The practice of medicine involves searching for answers to assist patients. It is supposed to revolve around taking an interest in healing the body and the overall well-being of the patient.

Looking back now, I can see clearly the shortcomings. Physicians are imprisoned with narrow thinking and overly specific, segmented information and views of the physiology of the human body, always looking at one part and not the part related to the whole. Plus, they never take the proper required time to evaluate or question the individual patient's progress, the true health progress. In fact, what are their evaluation methods for treatment and its success? Are they even aware if, indeed, they are using the most appropriate evaluation methods within their practice? If they are, are the methods and treatment continually assessed and modified to bring about the best result for that "individual?" Furthermore, are there sensible and appropriate evaluations of the patient when copious amounts of medicines are prescribed? In my case, medication after medication was prescribed and each time a new symptom suddenly turned up following its use. Why wasn't this a clue as to the disrupting effect the medication was having upon the body? Wasn't this a big red flag saying, "Wait; what is going on here?" They simply ignored these flags and were completely oblivious to them. They just prescribed and prescribed, for one symptom after another. It was drug/symptom, drug/symptom, continuing an impractical and vicious cycle. All the while, the poor body is trying to cope by compensating and re-adjusting its internal mechanisms just to sustain life. In support of my theory was the information I had just read about my medication the previous day when in the pharmacy. The long list of what the drug companies and traditional field of medicine say are "side-effects" are really "the effects the drugs have on your system." Also, each 'individual' is unique and these "effects" may be more or less pronounced, depending upon the specific makeup of that individual. One can even exhibit unusual effects not even mentioned about the drug. Could this be the reason for all my suffering with what seemed to be unrelated health challenges to my allergies? Could this also relate to all of the allergy injections I had received over the years? At this point it did seem plausible to me.

The following days were really rough for me. I was still completely shut down, still in shock, and emotionally feeling helpless. I could still barely get out of bed. I still felt, "Why go on?" I continued reciting my mantra over and over again. Then one of my sisters phoned me. She said she had just come from visiting with a college friend of hers. She didn't even recognize her; she looked absolutely fabulous. The last time she had seen her was almost a year prior. At that time her friend was ill, but did not know what was going on health-wise. My sister remembered how lifeless she looked, very grey with pale skin, the whites of her eyes almost black, and she had very dark circles under her eyes. She told my sister she suffered from extreme headaches and blackouts while she was traveling in Europe and had to come home. She saw a few top doctors in Los Angeles who did not help her. She then flew around the country to see doctors at the most prestigious medical institutions. Everyone told her there was nothing wrong with her and that she should seek some psychiatric assistance or some type of emotional therapy. She knew something was wrong with her health and that she was not crazy! She then came across a holistic practitioner, living and practicing in Los Angeles, who was from England. She went to see him and was absolutely intrigued with the way in which he went about unraveling her health mystery in a very short period of time. He was a warm, caring person and took a keen interest in her and her health. This was such a surprise to her, a complete one hundred and eighty degree turn from all the traditional doctors she had seen. He did a very long and extended history and intake with her; then he told her he believed she was being exposed to something very toxic and the symptoms she was suffering from were due to this toxicity. In just this initial visit and the next he pinpointed what it was. She was absolutely dumbfounded that the doctors she had seen across the country had never even asked a few simple questions, including ones about her work environment. This practitioner's approach was simple and thorough and just as his title described, "holistic." He began to work with her body, cleansing and nourishing, rebalancing over all. In the process, the toxic substances were expelled and discharged from her system and just as he had anticipated, her health was inherently being restored. In a short period of time she was feeling better and optimum health ensued. She told my sister she could not believe she needlessly suffered for all that time. My sister asked her for his phone number so that she could pass it along to me.

My sister finished her story about her friend and then said to me that I should arrange to see him because he might be able to help me. Well, in an instant a BIG emotional wall went up and I became very defensive. "Absolutely not," was my answer without even thinking about it. I began defending my conventional treatment that was now at the end of the road. I defended a future of living in an air-purified bubble! How funny is that? I actually commented to my sister, "What if I get worse faster?" In spite of all the insights that had come to me about my condition in the past few days, I was actually defending the doctors. All of a sudden I even believed I was not in such bad shape. I instantly became rock solid on my defensive grounds. My sister could not believe what she was hearing from me. She was baffled to say the least. She finally said to me, "The doctors say there is nothing more they can do for you; are you going to settle for that?" "Do you really want to live the rest of your life in an air-purified bubble?" "Do you really believe that is your future?" "There is nothing you have to lose in going to see this holistic practitioner." Hmm, I said to myself at that point, I could always go back to this downward spiral of suffering if he could not help me. She said she was calling herself to make an appointment for me. She insisted she would drag me there herself no matter what. God bless my sister for being so stern, blunt, and persistent and not letting me say "no." I **love** you, Madeleine! **Thank you too,** dad, my angel, for watching over me. You were right; "don't lose hope; we will find you help."

Resurrecting My Health

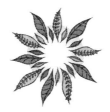

I went the next afternoon to see this holistic practitioner in his home office. I have to admit, and don't know why, that I was very scared. I had been seeing "medical doctors," believing they were solely concerned about my health and my well being; this is the most common assumption and we have been trained to accept it. I was conditioned to this. I was not sure what to expect from another type of practitioner with a different approach and medical training background. Again, looking back at that time, I never imagined myself getting better and being well. I was stuck, so focused on sickness and suffering and not feeling well that I never imagined things would change. I could not even comprehend a wellness path. I never mentally saw for myself a place of optimum health; how I would feel, who I would be. I was so comfortably uncomfortable with my sickness. A change was scary and would be a new way for me if I did get better. At this point, I was more fearful of the possibility of improving my health than remaining where I was, ultimately headed toward life in a bubble. It is amazing how we become conditioned to a particular way.

After ringing the bell, the practitioner opened the door. With a big warm smile he said "Welcome, love, come in and have a seat." Well this was quite different from any appointment I had had in the past. Wow, what a statement that was. I was also fascinated in that instant with his vibrant appearance. He was tall, had very healthy, glowing skin, and there was this radiant energy exuding from him. He had a delightful demeanor to match. I had no idea how my life was going to change from this point on. I filled out intake information for him and he began asking me questions. As we continued he began explaining allergies, from a holistic point of view. I would ask him some questions along the way about the other health challenges, a discussion would ensue, and every time his response made sense to me. In fact, to most things I had questioned the doctors about and never got an answer, he responded very eloquently. That's right. We had a discussion. He did not just tell me with a snide, arrogant look and then barely let me ask a question like the doctors who had been treating me. They just kept saying they knew and were not listening to what I was asking or describing to them about how crappy I really felt. I was being befriended by this practitioner. He was very interested in how I was feeling. No matter what I asked, it was important and he acknowledged me. He was amazingly supportive. I felt like he was standing in my shoes all along and experiencing what I had gone through all these years. He was discussing human physiology and how all our organ systems function together and communicate with each other. A wealth of additional physiological information was discussed. It was all making sense. I saw a new light; **I now had hope.** He wanted me to gain a new perspective in support of the path I would now take. He also wanted me to understand the more holistic approach and make sure it made sense to me. My mind was opening up to really seeing that I could get better.

In a short period of time with him, a wave of gratitude filled me. I began to feel blessed that I was even breathing and functioning at the level I was. I also felt blessed that someone actually seemed to truly care how I was feeling. Everything I discussed with him was significant, no matter what it was. The recognition again of how my body had been trying to rebalance was reinforced. I understood how my body was not getting what it needed to bring this about. All of my insights just previously realized were completely congruent to what he was discussing. The information supporting my theory over all was shining through. His explanations began with the fact that I had some weaker organ systems from early on. Since all of the major organ systems communicate and function in concert with each other, if there are a few that are weaker, tremendous strain is placed on the other organ systems, and complete balance within the body is disrupted. In my situation, the pollens and air environment surrounding me posed a threat to my health. They created major stress upon organ systems within my body and could not cope. Immediately, an analogy to this situation came to my mind that completely made sense. If a wagon filled with goods is to be pulled by a number of horses and one or two horses become fatigued or injured and cannot pull their weight any longer, great strain will be placed upon the other horses. Complete imbalance will result. The other horses will now have to work harder, will fatigue faster and they too may become injured in a shorter period of time. An even simpler analogy would be if you are driving and get a flat tire. If you attempt to keep driving, not only will that wheel structure wear out very quickly, but the other three wheels will be wearing unevenly. Tremendous strain will be placed upon these and other structures of the car. Over all, the whole car will become dysfunctional and out of balance in a short period of time. It will not be able to transport you anywhere!

With regard to my health, western treatment was based on a minute portion of my body that was reacting to the environment, desensitizing a population of cells known to react. Only a part of the "whole" physiological system was being addressed. Then medications entered to halt the multitude of symptoms my body responded with, again only addressing a part of the "whole." He did state that the numerous health challenges I had over the years were a sign that my body was moving away from regaining health, also attributing this to the effects of all the medications. Years of daily antihistamines, antibiotics, analgesics, the allergy serums, etc were degenerating my system and disrupting Homeostasis. They were not addressing the "root" of the cause, they were halting fragmented parts of the "whole" body's response. Additional factors included the fact that the medications were not completely being cleared from my system, a common problem for anyone taking prescription medications. This is due to the fact that all drugs have a half-life, a specific time they take to be broken down and eliminated from the system, lasting anywhere from days to weeks to months. I was medicating abundantly on a daily basis, thus making it even more difficult, virtually impossible, to completely clear the medications from my system at all. As a result my system was in a constant state of toxicity, eventually leading to over-acidity. How did my body respond? Not very well. My body moved toward a more severely imbalanced state. Naturally, my body did not like this state and began an uphill battle to manage this completely inharmonious situation. How could it even remotely try to accomplish this without the necessary tools it was missing? Plus, how could it accomplish this when it was being bombarded with medications that temporarily stopped symptoms, blocked and shut down *vital* physiological pathways, and completely interfered with the *operational intelligence* of the body? It could not accomplish this nor cope with the situation. The allergies got worse and the multitude of additional health challenges resulted from the constant assault of treatment. These health challenges included intestinal degeneration (often referred to as "leaky gut"), chronic Candida, adrenal fatigue, severe dehydration, general toxicity and over acidity (previously mentioned), severe headaches along with sinus pains, bladder and kidney problems, just to name a few. I was also having rebound effects from taking so many medications; the symptoms would disappear for a shorter and shorter duration of time after taking the medication and then rebound at an even more intense level.

Things were now beginning to make sense to me and the explanations followed through logically because the practitioner was looking at the body as a "whole." If I were to draw a diagram of my sickness path over the years it would match the explanations given.

He started to map out a treatment plan for me. He said it would take time, but I would notice improvements along the way. He encouraged full trust in my body knowing how to heal and not to get discouraged. Initially, it was crucial for me to cleanse my system. This would relieve a lot of my more immediate symptoms and challenges (i.e. severe kidney distress being the most recent). A combination of medicinal herbs, Homeopathic drainage formulas, and various fresh juice recipes, containing foods known to cleanse and nourish the liver and lymph system were a part of my regimen. We would then focus on nourishing organ systems, the regenerating phase, thus restoring my vital energy and homeostasis within my body. In my case, his approach was to incorporate herb food formulations, homeopathic formulas, more alkaline foods, alkaline/ionized water, meditation and deep breathing practices, and restorative energy techniques. He again stressed that I should not get discouraged. The healing path would be like peeling away layers of an onion. There would be times when some symptoms might return and resurface as my body cleansed, but the duration would not be like the original problems I had experienced. I might experience some fatigue, but this was also normal and due to cleansing. It would not be from feeling drained with a new specific health challenge like I had had over the years. I also might feel less energetic for a period of time as an enormous amount of energy would be required to rebuild and regenerate my health. When this happens, he advised, "listen to your body, love. Rest as much as you need to; don't over-exert yourself. You will notice improvements in spite of all this."

The fascinating thing about the human body is that when it gets what it needs and can utilize this, it will take immediate care to rebuild and rebalance the systems that are in the most dire, crucial state. Then it will move to other systems to rebuild and rebalance. It might go back and forth between systems, rebuilding and rebalancing, until proper over all balance is achieved and homeostasis is regained. **Patience** was needed he said with **encouragement.** This was magnificent; he was laying out the anticipated healing path my body would take. Never had the doctors I saw ever mentioned anything like this. I was now developing a complete sense of confidence in my body to regain health. Wow! What an absolutely amazing shift! I began seeing for myself that my body knew how to struggle to barely keep its balance for all these years and keep me alive. If it now got what it really needed and got rid of what it did not like (drugs, etc.), it would only know the way of health. This was fact, not a theory.

I faithfully followed the recommended plan he advised. In six months I began feeling better than I had in twenty years! I thought I was dreaming. Was I cured? No. However, the improvements were magnificent from cleansing and detoxifying alone in the first few months. It was a bit challenging over those six months, but I was very ill and, as he advised, had to be patient. I had been ill for twenty years and it had only been six months so far on a new course. Improvements surfaced along the way, slowly but surely even in the very beginning. This was affirming to me and kept me adhered to the journey. He stuck by my side very closely, answering questions and supporting my journey also. He expressed empathy when I was not feeling too good and was elated and joyful alongside me when I felt great. What incredible gifts I was receiving from my body along the way as well. More gratitude filled my soul. This was a completely different experience from all those years when the doctors said, "Just be patient." During that time, I never improved, just stayed the same, and then regressed. The doctors were not supportive, let alone even seeming to care. This time I noticed improvements every single day, even though they were minute at times. If symptoms resurfaced as he mentioned they would, I stuck with it and eventually reaped the rewards. I kept feeling better and better. Week by week I could feel my body getting rid of what it didn't want and getting what it needed. I slowly felt my body functioning more efficiently over all and balance being restored.

I then moved into the second six months of our treatment plan. I continued to be ecstatic about how good I was feeling. At times I was weary and apprehensive about possibly not sustaining this as in the past, having a period of improved health and then nose-diving down the other way. However, this time I was noticing shifts in my body I hadn't experienced before. My healing path was following that description of layers of an onion being peeled away. The health challenges that had come about more recently, just before this holistic path, were disappearing. Most recent symptoms were being shed; then my body began dealing with the next symptoms, then on to the next. For example, as my body cleansed and detoxified, my kidney and bladder issues began clearing up. This, as I mentioned, was the most recent challenge before beginning this healing path. With the renewed health in this area, my body could now focus on the next layer of cleansing, if needed, and regenerating other systems. The energy used to bring about health in this area could now be directed toward another area. My body could move forward toward optimizing health with even more support from other organ systems. At the same time, I was experiencing my body's core inner intelligence to re-establish true balance. With homeostasis emerging, my body was now standing healthier. The improvements I was experiencing were noticeably stronger, as though my body were building a new core foundation to support itself. I had never experienced this over the previous years, let alone sustaining any level of health like this. The path was getting easier and easier and the healing was even more pronounced. I was improving in a logarithmic fashion. Now I was completely rooted in faith, my body fully capable of restoring its health. Symptom after symptom was disappearing, one organ system after the other was strengthening.

As the practitioner mentioned, there were days when my energy was very low, but I could hear his words in my head saying, "Listen to your body, love." I did listen to my body and let it relax. In fact, some days I was so tired I could barely lift my arms and legs to get out of bed. However, this did not last for long and in a short period of time following, I would notice my energy and stamina improving. This was right in line with what he had discussed with me. As my healing path evolved, the focus on my allergies and not feeling well were diverted toward the positive improvements and feeling well. I would then notice that my allergies had diminished significantly.

Weeks without all the allergic reactions and symptoms were turning into a few months. I was able to venture outside with more and more confidence that steadily kept growing. My whole emotional outlook stayed positive. The symptoms that had cleared over this time did not return, thus demonstrating that my body was balancing and doing well. I continued following up with the practitioner, sticking to the plan and being faithful in my commitment. He was excited for me and so pleased that I was feeling better. The next year I felt even better. My allergies were falling by the wayside and my health was regenerating at a phenomenal rate. I was able to be active in my daily life, pursuing activities I was deprived of over the years. Just being able to go outside and breath without the fears of all those years was spectacular!

One day, the following year, I was on a walk and went up a hilly street to a fire road. Without even thinking about any allergy condition, I walked along the road for a bit and then turned around to look at the view of the city off in the distance. I could see a huge layer of smog. I also noticed that there were weeds and various shrub plants surrounding me everywhere. Some were so tall they had grown up to shoulder height. I closed my eyes, took in a few deep breaths, and then opened my eyes. What a revelation. I realized I was standing face to face with what previously haunted me, weeds, plants, and nature, and was breathing in my former vicious enemy, the air. We were now allies. I had never felt better in my life! I shouted out loud to my body, "we did it!"

As time went on I continued to remain vibrantly healthy. I supported my new health however much I could. As the years went by, it became increasingly more difficult for me to even remember how I used to feel. I had no idea how I coped on a daily basis for the twenty years I suffered. It felt like that was literally another person. True resurrection had commenced.

It had now been about three years in total, only three years in time that my health had been restored compared to the twenty that I suffered through. I had a new best friend and life-long companion who had stuck by me during the sick years and every day of the regenerative, healing years, my body. Wasn't that fascinating?

As I have shared my story with others over the years, the responses of people have fascinated me. The most interesting of the responses has been, "It took you that long to get better, three years?" I always smile and say, "Compared to twenty years of ill health, that is no time at all. Isn't the body truly amazing?" After my response they always stop and ponder for a few minutes and say, "I never thought of it that way."

When the body gets what it truly needs, in support of all of its physiological processes, the path toward optimum health is always shorter than the time it takes the body to manifest and exhibit the symptoms of chronic health conditions. *What an evolutionarily extraordinary organism the human body is.*

**"Thou in me art divine inspiration,
revelation, *faith*, and illumination."**

From this point on, my thoughts about the human body, health and healing were transformed. I was inspired, had new revelations, and a new path had been brilliantly illuminated for me. I shifted my professional health related background from clinical biomedical research into a holistic path to assist others on their journey.

Resurrection of Western Medicine

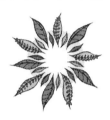

am not completely against western medicine. However, I proved the doctors wrong. Millions of people all around the world, just like myself, prove doctors' predictions wrong every day. The working innate intelligence of the human body, along with proper assistance, rises above internal health imbalances and challenges, bio-chemically restructures itself, and ultimately restores *Homeostasis*, thus perpetuating life. The "initial grim medical predictions" we hear all the time are obliterated. We need to emotionally bond to and embrace this body intelligence and know that if we work in alignment with our body and its intelligence, this will facilitate and re-direct physiological processes back to their normal *Homeostatic* state. Thus, improved health will inherently ensue. Western medicine afforded me slight symptom relief initially and epinephrine was my lifesaver for an unexpected acute, severe, systemic allergic response, provided it could be administered within the narrow time frame to halt the deadly response.

However, western medicine kept me ill and induced further severe health challenges, causing me to suffer for an unnecessarily long period of time over all. The innate intelligence of the body and its relentless, physiological efforts to maintain *Homeostasis* were completely ignored and grossly unrecognized due to the mindset of western medicine. Only symptoms were addressed and suppressed, but not the underlying root causes of these symptoms, their relationship to one another, nor their relationship or association to my initial health challenge. An unbelievably simple concept which could have been addressed was whether many of the symptoms that arose over the years could actually have been induced by the medications prescribed. There were no attempts to deduce their cause or what role these symptoms played in my expanded suffering as time went on.

So what is the current mindset of western medicine? There have been miraculous advances in some areas of medicine over the years (surgery techniques, etc.); however, in general, medicine has been failing us in a *grandiose* manner. As medical practices have become more specialized, drug addicted, and devoid of compassion over the years, the gaps for creating true health and wellbeing have widened. The "whole" has been fragmented into many pieces. As medicine continues to become more specialized and less personalized, approaching a pace faster than the speed of light, the gaps will widen even further. Western medicine views a particular body part, organ system, or function in *complete* oblivion to the fact that it is a "part" of the "whole" human body. The "whole body" itself will not even be considered. The ability to relate the "part" to the "whole" will soon be non-existent.

Medical training, in its early stages, orients the mind to view organ systems and their biochemical processes as separate units, functioning on their own. The orchestration of biochemical reactions and processes in one system and how they interact and direct other systems are rarely emphasized and followed in the learning process. The basic cascade, flow, and constant interaction of these working principles are what the body uses to maintain *Homeostasis* (balance) and to restore and achieve health within the organism. If in the educational process the mind is not trained to follow these working principles within the body in this manner, it will not be able to recognize and comprehend these working principles and interacting relationships; thus, essential premises relating to health restoration will be overlooked. Even the most simple premises for health restoration are overlooked. Medical training breezes over valuable foundational physiological and anatomical information related to the functioning of the human body and processes by which the body moves toward imbalances and presents illness. At the same time, the innate working intelligence and physiological truths the body presents of how it heals are not logically addressed or recognized. Thus, the disconnection of the "part" to the "whole" begins. Now add into the picture the utilization of high tech analysis. This is useless if it is not carefully molded around the human body's organic holistic functioning, and personally interfaced with the individual involved. There is a rush to the finish line looking only at symptoms, attempting to obliterate them no matter what the paying price. Costly drugs, and/or surgery are employed which are not only very costly to us and to the price of healthcare we pay in general, but commonly jeopardize our health further, leaving many in a much more dire health situation than before any treatment started. Another most disturbing component of western medicine today is that even if we express to our doctors that we feel healthy and well overall and an exam shows this for the most part, they are relentlessly luring us into believing we are not optimally well.

They scrutinize tests looking for a slight open door upon analysis through which they can emphasize the necessity to prescribe medication. More and more these recommendations to take medications are for life! Plus, the age of the patient to which they are prescribed is getting younger and younger, placing more lives at risk and for longer periods of time. This ensures that the drugs "life span" will increase, being prescribed to even more people for a longer period over one's life. The doctor's are not, however, working alone here. Their strongest ally and the backbone to this luring structure are the drug companies. In a most deceitful manner, the drug companies have created false health threats, employing fear and panic tactics directed toward us to brainwash us into believing that we absolutely are in need of their drugs. In fact, our *life* is literally dependent upon them. At the same time, the drug companies have been enticing doctors to perpetuate this cycle by offering them lavish kickbacks and perks of all kinds, including the placement of doctors on drug company payrolls, often with salaries that are greater than their medical practices produce. This, in turn, has kept doctors in a tyrannical hold thereby molding their practices into justified, glorified drug dispensaries. All of these actions have occurred at the brutal expense of our health, wellbeing, and lives.

> **"And we have made of ourselves living cesspools,
> and driven doctors to invent names for our diseases."**
>
> **—Plato**

As the body moves toward a state of illness, it lays down a map of how it got to that stage and also lays down a time frame for us. This map also contains treasures and abundant clues illuminating the path back toward health and wellness. A multitude of problems has arisen within the teachings of western medicine due to the fact that the skills to properly read the map in either direction have not been developed. The lack of these skills leads to failure to recognize *key* signs and clues the body gives. Western medical training has strayed far off the course of teaching how to recognize these *key* signs and clues, then process this information in relationship to basic human structure and function. This, in turn, makes it difficult to interpret the directions the map reveals for which way to proceed to restore health and wellness. It is scary and quite alarming that a majority of physicians today who specialize are not even aware of some of the basic structure-function relationships of human physiology outside of their specialty. How can they fully understand a specific area of the body without even knowing the neighboring organs and structures and their interrelated functions (part to whole)? If you need to have the radiator in your car replaced, the mechanic must know how to detach the hoses that connect to the radiator. This is a given for the mechanic to even do his job. He must then take out the radiator, replace it, reattach the main hoses to the new radiator and make sure all is mechanically working properly; otherwise the radiator is useless in the functioning of the car. The radiator (part) cannot perform its function just sitting under the hood of the car detached from the workings of the *whole* rest of the mechanical parts.

We, as patients, are also responsible for western medicine's downfalls. We have been trained to follow the doctor's prescribed course without questioning. We completely relinquish our health and responsibility for how we feel into the hands of someone else. We have become accustomed to expect drugs from the doctor, our quick fix. We eagerly take the medications in spite of really knowing why and we do not inquire about the effects they have on our body. When these effects arise, we just accept them and accommodate. We can literally feel horrible (I most certainly did) but never say a word to "the doctor." We do not actively listen to our body and too often if we know something is not right, we are afraid to question the "professional" for they are the "all mighty" one. In turn, these patterns of ours train the doctors to continue on the same course. This leads us all down the wrong paths, collectively fueling the misinterpretation of the map the body lays down (how health challenges progressed) along with the treasures and clues (how to restore health and wellness).

We need to take a proactive role in our health and wellbeing. You, the individual, know your body best. If we give up the responsibility of how our body feels, through ignoring it, being unaware, or giving this responsibility to someone else, like the doctor, we jeopardize our health even further. The illogical thinking is that this situation makes it easier to regain health. This could not be further from the truth. Giving up ownership of how we feel brings about greater difficulty in remedying the situation. The human body is a "gift" of life and along with that comes the "gift" of taking care of our body. If we give up this magical "gift," we give up the blessing to enjoy a vibrant, healthy life. So how do we embrace these "gifts" so we can enjoy life to its fullest? Invest time into learning basic principles about how your body functions along with simple principles of how to take care of it. The information you master, no matter how comprehensive it may be, is a pot of gold at your fingertips.

It is *essential* that we inform ourselves about how our own bodies intelligently operate and the basics of how they function, and then continually add knowledge to this repertoire by learning the foundational support we can provide it. Just as we learn to speak or walk, we must learn about our bodies. As we proceed in the educational process, we will automatically begin to learn how to listen to our bodies through their actions, shifts, and symptoms, how to read the maps it displays, and how we can respond in a physiologically compatible manner with its inherent intelligence. If we are seeking a doctor's help, we must communicate and work *with* him/her whether they like it or not, conveying the pertinent observations we make about our body. You, the patient, always know your body best! You, the patient, should be actively involved in treatment. Your descriptions, questions, and feedback should only be welcomed by any practitioner. In fact, this is the opportune time to learn and empower yourself with additional knowledge about your body. Ask questions and more questions. It is a magnificent blessing to know how the human body functions, let alone our own body. At the same time, this is part of the practitioners job to educate.

You, the individual, know your body best. If we dodge this essential aspect and move away from being aware of how our bodies feel, even giving this responsibility up to someone else, including the doctors, we jeopardize our health even further. The illogical thinking is that these situations make it easier to regain health. This could not be further from the truth because if we become challenged with any health problems, it will be more difficult to remedy the situation. We will have abandoned the gift that comes with life, taking care of our bodies, and will have discarded the opportunity to know our bodies, along with important tools to guide us back on the path of health. If we just give up this magical gift to someone who is not ourselves, we have abandoned the treasures of health and have destroyed that roadmap leading us back to wellness.

It is, however, *never* too late to gain the upper hand and turn things around. It is *never* too late to begin a new journey, reorienting ourselves in the direction of adopting optimum health and wellness in our lives. Too many people give up all their power to doctors of western medicine, completely ignoring the fact that it is *their own body.* When this happens, the door is wide open for too many health disasters to occur. One foregoes the inherent gift we possess—the inherent intelligence of our own body to be guided back to health.

**"Break down the walls of Jerico -
free ourselves of the oppressive Pharohs"**

—Biblical reference

Symptom, symptom, symptom is the focus, for the most part, of western medicine, while the patient becomes trained in focusing on the quick symptom removal or, more accurately, symptom "masking," and palliative care. How is this even remotely supposed to achieve a health level among us?

For example, it absolutely baffles me that without a simple, proper bacterial culture, doctors prescribe antibiotics. Then, if the individual does not improve because he/she does not have a bacterial infection and the doctor does not know that, more antibiotics are prescribed. If the condition still does not improve, even more medicines are prescribed. Look at what one is faced with now: the creation of both physical and monetary deficits. Our body pays a hefty price. The repeated doses of antibiotics have adverse affects upon our system, including the destruction of the delicate health of our digestive system (leading quickly to immune system dysfunction), the first step toward manifesting profound imbalances within the body. Now the original health challenge is present and new challenges arise. Back to the doctors we will go and they will look only at the original problem. If they just attempt to treat this, the secondary health challenges will continue to mount, creating more internal imbalances. The body will manifest a greater number of challenges along with abundant new symptoms in an attempt to keep it alive. Remember, *Homeostasis* is the goal. If doctors are still unsuccessful in treating the first problem, round and round we will go. We go hopping right onto the merry-go-round. Wee! **Sick care system here we come**! I was on that ride for twenty years. Now, here come the financial costs. They include medications, doctors' visits, additional possible costly procedures, and valuable personal and work time lost. *Most importantly, we suffer!* What about our sanity? What price can we place on these losses?

On a broader scale relating to the example above, if the over-prescribing of antibiotics continues, we are directing bacterial pathogens to mutate and become resistant to these life-saving substances. If we do in fact need antibiotic treatment at some point and it does not work, then what? A cocktail of drugs? Hopefully that will work and if not, we are faced with a more serious health crisis and a more costly solution. The truth is we might not live at all. This situation is already occurring; if we don't begin to shift direction, we are headed toward a more destructive path.

Doctors give drugs of which they know little, into bodies, of which they know less, for diseases of which they know nothing at all.

—Voltaire

The fact is we are NOT feeling better and benefiting at large from what western medicine purports it can do for our health and should be accomplishing. In fact, its shortcomings have contributed to rising healthcare costs, promoting sickness, sustaining dis-ease, and creating abundant avoidable needless suffering. We are NOT paying for health care, we are paying for sick care. **We continue to pay into a sickness system not a wellness system.** In order to effectively restructure the system, "**wellness**" needs to be the focus and we must be involved in that demand. Western medicine needs this complete re-structuring. Centuries ago, a split and divergence of philosophies surrounding health practices and medicine evolved—a symptom vs. holistic approach. The word "medicine" has its roots in the Latin word "medicina," meaning "the art of healing." In classical Greek medicine, health was a matter of balance within the body, whereas disease was understood as an imbalance of the body (or at that time an imbalance in the bodily fluids, called "humors"). This balance could be restored by a medicus--alleviating, curing, and preventing further imbalances, thus restoring over all health and wellbeing. Those medicine professionals carried out their skill with feeling and compassion, a "good bedside manner" as we know it. Now is the time to circle back to the heart of what the human body's central functional needs are when *Homeostasis* is in crisis. What is medicine's purpose? What is at the center of its educational philosophy? Who are we attracting into the profession? How can we devise a comprehensive system to include the multitude of more holistically oriented modalities and practices that can address more individual needs? A good start is to first accurately define health and wellness and to embrace, as mentioned, the extraordinary intelligence of the body. The definition of health is not the suppression of one symptom while numerous others arise, creating greater health challenges in time than initially. Keeping people on medications (many more toxic and harmful than the initial illness) and expanding them to an exorbitant number for more and more people for life, is not creating wellness. This is still sickness and dis-ease. The approach of knocking out one or two symptoms with drugs, while a host of other drug induced symptoms arise, then treating these with more drugs which in turn create more side effects is not only insanity but worthless for creating wellness. Yet, the profession claims the patient is doing better and "well" over all. Western medicine should observe sickness, but relative to wellness. As medicine treats a part, is it contributing to the over all expansion of wellness—part related to whole? Let us not lose sight of the fact that we are dealing with human lives, with feelings, sensitivity, and emotions. Now we also have to do our part. We have to be compelled to master our own wellness. If our health is compromised and we do not feel better and we accept this, we are fueling the fire. If we are pursuing western treatments and do not feel better and ignore possible new symptoms without saying anything, and adjusting to debilitating drug effects on our bodies, then we are adding to this defective system and keeping it dysfunctional. We must ignite internal compassion and inspiration to forge forth towards body balance and true health.

We would benefit greatly from some creative incentives as well. Here is a proposed theory: while we get money refunds on our taxes, savings benefits on auto insurance and other related policies, and earn interest on money deposited in the bank, I believe we should receive abundant credits and refunds on health insurance for taking charge of our health and our being well. In ancient times in China, healers were not paid (compensated) if they did not keep people well. Perhaps we should receive a portion of payments back if we are still sick after medical treatment over a reasonable amount of time. Our suffering is worth time and money as well. At present, there is absolutely NO incentive for a wellness path or for western medicine to get us well and keep us that way. This might be one way to motivate doctors and the many people who are continuing on completely destructive health paths, even bringing their children along. Many are not consciously awake to the destructive patterns they have developed; however, sadly, many are aware but do not take even a small step to make the changes which can literally save their own or a loved ones life. These incentives should be available to practitioners as well. Maybe this would impart the motivation to review their education, philosophies, and actions and to go within themselves to convert robotic treatment actions, emotional desensitization, and immunity to the patient's progress. They would then proceed back into comprehensive, artistic, individualized care with sensitivity and compassion for the living organism that is struggling to regain a healthful balance. Both parties should be taking part in the joyful journey to wellness and everyone should be enjoying the treasures of health and wellbeing.

Education is another way to foster an appreciation for the bodies that are ours. It is perplexing that we spend numerous years in school learning a vast amount of required information. Virtually no time is spent learning about how our bodies function; how to nourish and nurture them, and how to take optimum care of ourselves. This should logically come first. How do we expect to function in general, let alone learn and contribute our gifts to the universe, if we are not even given the tools to keep ourselves vibrantly healthy? I am still trying to sort this one out. Can you?

Mastering Wellness

Medicine and Healing are an ART

We have lost the **ART** of healing within modern western medicine.

The skill and knack of the artistry no longer prevails. Ingenuity has evaporated. The perspectives have been severely distorted. The concept of looking at a part functionally related to the whole organism has completely vanished. The systematic use of common sense, basic reasoning, and a holistic oversight over all has been replaced with irrational, narrow-minded, robotic, often inaccurate information, and overly specialized ways.

Medicine has lost the *essence* of what health and wellness truly are. It has lost the *essence* of assisting in the creation of a Masterpiece—an individual, whom after treatment and care, is not just free of a few symptoms, even after dealing with resulting abundant new symptoms, but free of dis-ease and full of vitality and color representing true wellness.

You are the **MASTER** artist of your health. You are the one in charge. If your body is the canvas upon which an absolute masterpiece can be created, you are the sole director. Step back and look at your canvas--your body. Become a keen and objective observer in tune with how you are feeling. Constructively observe with kindness and care; evaluate your present state, just as you would observe a most spectacular art masterpiece. Begin obtaining knowledge about the health concerns or challenges you have observed and you are dealing with. Spend some time reviewing the symptoms you have. Have you always felt this way or were you feeling healthy and well at some point? Try to make a diagram depicting the path your body has taken to wind up in this state. Fully engage yourself in the process. Write down any thoughts or questions that come to your mind, no matter how insignificant they may seem to you. As you take an active role in the process, gain a variety of perspectives. You will be able to work with these as you begin your journey of creating your masterpiece of health.

Remember, you are the **MASTER** artist of your health.

Begin learning about the various issues you have now observed. Do some research including more holistic explanations and let yourself explore in order to gain a wider perspective. Formulate questions about the information you obtain. If you are currently being treated by a doctor and are not satisfied, don't be afraid to ask questions—it is your right! In fact, ask lots and lots of questions. Immunize yourself against any opposing intimidation. It is **YOUR BODY**! You are fully capable of understanding any information presented to you with some guidance and support. Doctors are supposed to educate the patient and learn from them as well. You can change your path or add on to your treatments at any stage; any time is the appropriate time. Look to people who have been where you are and have regained health. What healing options did they choose? Look toward people whom you know, even including family, who are well and can share what they do or even become a mentor for you. Share what you have found out with these people or others, work together. Ask questions, discuss, converse with others, again gaining additional perspectives. ***Don't give up.*** As you collect information, take time to digest it and analyze it. Find someone to assist you if you need help understanding what you have gathered. Too often, especially when it comes to prescription medications, major procedures and treatments (such as surgery or chemotherapy, etc.), we feel pressured or rushed into making a decision and do not take the time to evaluate or process it fully. Again, if needed, find someone who can assist you with explanations if you do not fully understand the condition or treatment options. Allow yourself time, as long as you need, to sit with the various options. Check into more holistic approaches you may have found if you have not already considered this, or into complementing avenues in support of more traditional medical treatment.

Now, like the artist who studies various techniques within the field (e.g. painting or sculpting, etc.), begin your wellness journey by gathering knowledge about various healing practices. Begin studying the related information. There is a wealth of various healing practices available for you to choose from to address your health concerns. You do not have to settle for just one of these. Like the master artist, mindfully choosing an array of colors to work with, even combining them to create ingenious, unique, distinctive colorful blends, you can pick and choose a variety of healing practices and modalities, blending them together for your individual condition(s). The foundational functioning of the human body is the same from person to person, so certain options and modalities are effective for everyone at certain basic levels; however, there will be additional ones that are needed for one person's health but not others. Some people may need additional practices at a different time than another or some may not need additional assistance at all. Just as no two works of art are ever the same, each individual may need additional fine-tuning assistance to achieve optimum health goals. The paths may be different at any one point for different people, but all the work will lead to the same place—***wellness***.

If you begin with a particular method(s) and you improve somewhat or not as much as you anticipate in a reasonable amount of time, step back and re-evaluate. Have you improved a great deal in one area and not in another or have you improved mildly in many areas? How long have you been working along this avenue? Don't be afraid to stop and reassess. However, over all, don't stop the momentum of your original intent of putting yourself in motion toward optimum health. ***Keep focused on the finished creation, the masterpiece—feeling vibrantly well on a consistent basis.*** Artists might spend a great deal of time on one particular area of a painting or sculpture and then shift to another area as they feel the need. They will use their intuition to guide themselves to the areas that need work until the piece is balanced and harmonious. As the master artist, give yourself the freedom to be guided in this fashion too while seeking that which supports your body's natural physiological processes.

As you begin to feel even the slightest bit better with regard to your health, your body will intelligently begin guiding you further along the divine right path. You will automatically begin to become aware of this and hone into the signals your body gives you. Begin asking for what you feel you need; you will be guided to the right answers. It is at this point that you want to fully embrace the *brilliance of your body* and its amazing capabilities. Trust, faith, and patience are your partners. The body knows what true health is if you keep steering it to what it needs for balance. *Foster a loving internal bond with the physiological brilliance of your body.*

TRUST in your abilities to understand the basic functioning of your body and how the health challenge(s) or condition(s) might be affecting the normal balance. Again, seek assistance with this if you need it. As the master artist you will gain experience in seeking that which will support your body's natural balance. Take action and keep the process in motion. Even if the steps you take are very tiny in the beginning, in time they will all add up. As your body begins healing, you will become excited to see it continually compound the positive results, creating more and more health at a steady rate. Consistency will be worth its weight in gold.

Priming for the Masterpiece

Artists know that preparation and priming are keys to laying down the foundation from which a masterpiece can be created. No matter what state of health you are currently in, there are several basic areas of preparing and priming to focus on, thus laying down the foundation for your masterpiece of wellness. Once you set your plan in motion, no matter where you choose to begin, your new wellness path will be illuminated. **Contrary** to what most people think and are advised, mainly the idea that one needs to make numerous and massive changes all at once, you can and may need to begin taking infinitesimal *but consistent steps*. Once you begin taking action in one area--***open sesame***--everywhere you turn, doors will magically open, guiding you along the path to renewed health and wellness. This path will effortlessly begin unfolding before you. *You do not have to know exactly how but know it will, as that is the way of the universe when you put your desire into motion. Be ready, open, aware, and expect what you believe are*

absolute miracles to come your way and the subtle ways in which they appear and might cross your path. Nothing is too good to be true! For example, you may, out of the blue, come across key information related to your condition or a modality that others have benefited from. You may meet a stranger during your outings, in the market for instance, who shares pertinent information or an experience relating to your new path. You may even meet a complete stranger who has dealt with the same ailment or a similar one or some other health challenge and is now vibrantly well and has an offering for you. A friend or family member may enlighten you with some unexpected information or direction for you. There are an infinite number of blessings that will appear and ways in which they will touch your life and wellness journey and will come to you at the *exact appropriate time.* Bring yourself to the highest spiritual place of expecting events and support that will lead you toward a healthy and well "you." You attract what you think. As you progress on your journey and create the *expectant* mindset, you will begin to feel very special, as if you are the most important person. You are! ***You are worthy of feeling the best that you can feel.*** God is recognizing your efforts and your path will continue to be supported. ***Divine wellness is meant for you.*** Feeling good, both physically and emotionally, will also connect us with our highest divine good and purpose.

I continuously experienced angelic guidance and direction like this along my wellness journey. Also, even though my father had passed on, he was frequently with me, my advocate, an angel still present at my side. Once I chose to work with the holistic practitioner, feeling more safe and cared for, every day was filled with blessings, miracles in fact, in support of my wellness path. I will always be grateful for all of them, especially this one: after every appointment with my holistic practitioner, when I returned home at about the same time, I would look out my kitchen window, praying that my condition would improve and continue to get better and better. At the same time, an adorable red-breasted bird would sit, facing me, on the telephone wire stretching across from the pole to the building. It would start vigorously singing and belting its voice out so loud I would start to laugh. I even thought the bird might pass out! Just when I did laugh, it would stop for a minute and stare right at me, give a few loud chirps, then begin its tune again. God, an angel, my father, however I wanted to interpret it, was a **blessing**, the universe validating my new path.

Once you set your intention of creating wellness and take some form of action, the process will automatically be set in motion and continue. Now, *get out of your own way* and don't let others interfere with your journey either. As Newton's first law of motion states—every object in a state of uniform motion tends to remain in that state of motion unless an external force is applied to it. Immunize yourself against the strongest forces, the ego-defeating part of our psyche which will try to con you into believing you cannot accomplish that which your heart desires. It will lash out with every excuse from being difficult, a struggle, doubtful, fearful, resentful, or angry to feeling sad, lonely, and undeserving, to mention just a few. Beware! Also, beware of the ego con artist in others who may have already bought into those defeating beliefs. They, too, will try every avenue to sabotage, destroy or inhibit your wellness journey, projecting all kinds of inhibiting forces upon you. Others may think they are being supportive when, in fact, they are subconsciously trying to sabotage you. Just continue in motion, remaining calm and focused on *your* masterpiece of health; you will gain productive momentum and you will manifest the accomplishment you desire.

With regard to your body's physiology, the new actions you begin taking will set into motion new tools for your body to work with. Remember, your body knows **only** what optimum health is. You are still **ALIVE**. As you begin *congruently* supporting the working intelligence of its physiology and biochemistry, it will know where to begin its work and how to regenerate its health. From one cell to another to another, Newton's first law of motion will again take place, but now on a cellular level. From one cell to another, to another, to another, each will be restructuring and restoring its optimum functioning. This momentum will continue to build as even more cells are enlisted. All these cells will now be healthier and begin interacting and communicating more effectively with each other, eventually restoring your body's inherent *Homeostasis*. Continue taking action, *infinitesimal* steps if needed, keep focused and don't stop, even if you do not notice immediate improvements. We need to remember that every cell has its own life-cycle time. Now you need to begin raising your mental and emotional level of expectancy for your body to repair and renew itself. You need to send an internal message of confidence to your cells: confidence in their ability to utilize the intelligence and re-build cellular health and balance. Now you need faith, faith to fuel the expectancy of improved wellness.

So many people, once they decide to make new health promoting changes, become extremely impatient. I know; I was in this position at first also. The mind says, "Okay, I made the decision and I took some action; its been five days and I don't feel better; I guess nothing is working." Maybe it has been two weeks or even a month but you are still frustrated. I know what this feels like and it is another angle the conning ego part of the psyche is trying to strike you with. This is when we need to step back and become an objective observer of ourselves. Was the

Mona Lisa painted in a few days? It is absolutely amazing how one can experience less than optimum wellness and dis-ease for a very long period of time, but become so impatient when making more holistic changes or adjusting one's previous so-called health path. We become upset and frustrated with our bodies. We want everything to improve now, even yesterday. We are quick to dismiss the logical, positive effects that will result from newly introduced wellness actions, let alone subtle changes that are brought about by the body at various stages of healing. In fact, we may misinterpret these changes if we are not fully engaged in the process our body needs or do not learn about how it holistically restores health along the way. For example, your body may be in dire need of cleansing out toxins. You experience cleansing symptoms and misinterpret this as a new health challenge. This is very interesting. It is strange that people are very patient and understanding when they receive conventional treatments and don't feel better immediately. Over and over, people go to their doctors without hesitating or questioning for the most part the progress of treating their health condition or imbalance. Day after day, month after month, year after year, we trot back to the doctor, feeling just as bad or, more often, much worse. We never question but just do as we are told. Then there is the prescription medication dilemma. Medications are prescribed and taken, and either the condition does not improve right away or the condition improves but your body feels worse, either immediately or over time from the side-effects of the medication. We just follow the orders to fill the prescription and take the medications because the doctor tells us it will help, or we continue the medications and feel awful because we are told we will get used to the side-effects, no matter how severe they are (yes, they are worse than how we felt originally and are often deadly!).

In support of resurrecting your health and creating your wellness masterpiece, **now** is the time to embrace your body. Even the most subtle, minute positive shift that can easily be taken for granted is monumental improvement on a cellular level. **Now** is the time to express gratitude and love for the body's amazing capabilities and brilliance. **Now** is the time to back your new wellness journey with faith. You are still **ALIVE**--don't give up now! You must **now** embrace your body's own timing for healing. It is your body's timing, not what your expected timing is. Your body inherently knows what action to take and in what part of the body to take it when you incorporate healing principles that are *congruent* to the physiology and biochemistry of the body. First, you may be experiencing very unpleasant symptoms that you want to go away. However, your body may need to repair tissues and organs not directly related to those symptoms before it can relieve the ones you are expecting at first. Whatever part of the body needs dire healing attention, the body will attend to first. Its intelligence will immediately begin directing cellular functioning in the most appropriate area. At the microscopic level, this is often a different place than what we may expect or believe needs assistance. We are often not even aware, at the microscopic level, of the imbalances and challenges that cells of a particular organ or tissue have been struggling with. However, your body knows what needs repair and restoration first, in order for it to re-establish Homeostasis within.

The human body is magnificent! Yes, for the most part it is complex beyond comprehension; however, when it receives the proper biocompatible tools it needs to repair, regenerate, and heal, it will take them and turn dis-ease into health-ease.

Choose to resurrect your health. Set your wellness journey into motion **now.** Create a viable understanding of the following information and take an empowering action from one or all of these simple, basic, fundamental, foundational areas. Your masterpiece is now underway. Enjoy the creative process.

Foundations for Mastering Wellness

Foods

The body is made up of trillions of microscopic cells, each of which requires various nutrients to support their structure and functioning. They also require immense amounts of energy to keep them active and working at their peak. Health and wellness are *vitally* dependent upon these factors. In fact, **LIFE** is dependent upon these factors. There is one basic fundamental question that is completely overlooked by the majority of people and most surprisingly and sadly by the majority of western health professionals, those supposedly here "to take care of our health." That is, **why do we eat? Why do we need to eat food at all?** Once you become enlightened and aware of the answer and foster an appreciation of it by befriending the extraordinary functions of your body's microscopic cells and what they need to thrive and optimally survive, and once you know what foods can provide, your journey will *instantly* become easier.

Foods provide the essential nutrients our cells need to build their structures and support their functions. Food is also fuel, fuel for these trillions of microscopic cells making up your extraordinary body. Each and every one of these cells requires utilizable nutrients obtained from foods. Without proper foods (generally classified into carbohydrates, proteins, and fats), cells will not receive adequate amounts of utilizable nutrients. As a result, cells begin to deteriorate and dysfunction (cellular structures and molecules of life become defective), become more susceptible to pathogenic attack (viruses, etc.), and function at a less than optimal capacity. They will even die off. As a result, it should not be surprising that dis-ease and numerous health challenges will ensue at some point in time. Cells are basically little factories, continuously breaking down molecular structures into basic building block components (catabolism) and reforming molecular structures with these basic building blocks (anabolism) when needed to maintain their proper structure and function and to provide the necessary components to continuously work synergistically, making necessary adjustments when needed, either individually or collectively with other cells of the body. It is imperative that cells continuously receive proper *life-sustaining* nutrients to keep these processes going. The absolute *exquisite beauty* of human physiology is the synergy and ability to easily and rapidly adjust when needed. This inherent and autonomous working principle is known as *Homeostasis.* This is the process our body uses to actively maintain stable, balanced, steady-state conditions necessary for survival. A healthy state is one that is maintained by this principle, *Homeostasis,* the process of constantly adjusting biochemical and physiological pathways whenever needed through collective coordinated responses, thereby bringing about balance.

Cells also require immense amounts of energy to function efficiently and effectively and to survive. Thus, they not only continuously and masterfully transform molecular components making up foods into essential components required for their structures and functions, but also derive utilizable energy (metabolically generated in the form of the molecule ATP) to maintain their existence and overall functioning. The energy produced is used to do work, specific work, depending on the type of cell. With the essential nutrients and adequate amounts of energy, cells will thrive. They will continue to be healthy and vibrant while carrying out their work, and when needed, they will be able to duplicate or divide themselves through the process known as *mitosis,* whereby old cells are continuously replaced by new cells at a varying rate, depending on the cell type. The healthier the cell is before it divides, the healthier the duplicate new cell will be. If cells are depleted and malfunctioning prior to their dividing, their duplicates can only be of lesser health. This new generation of cells (depleted/malfunctioning) will eventually go through mitosis as well and the new cells will again be of lesser health and function at a diminished capacity. Thus, we can see that we will have a dilution effect of cellular health as more and more cells are duplicated over time. As time goes on and the majority of cells in a particular organ are replaced with depleted, malfunctioning cells, the whole organ system's capacity to carry out its function will be compromised. The cells' individual and collective capacity to maintain health will be greatly diminished, even severely damaged. In time, millions of cells will be operating at a fraction of their capacity, some not even functioning at all. The maintenance of normal internal stability achieved through the multitude of coordinated responses of organ systems, *Homeostasis*, will be destroyed. These cells will no longer be able to adjust their functional capacity to re-establish this *Homeostatic* balanced state. Now, let me ask you this: don't you want your cells to be successively healthier upon dividing? Don't you want them to thrive and be functioning only at peak performance to maintain *Homeostasis*, the regulatory process of life, or do you want them to become depleted, dysfunctional, uncoordinated and eventually die? I certainly hope you want the former scenario. I know I do!

Another core component related to knowing why the foods we eat (and what we drink) are important to health is that they shape the *internal body terrain*, which in turn supports and actively contributes to the life-sustaining process of *Homeostasis*. This *internal terrain*, mainly known as the pH environment (acid-alkaline/base environment), is the *internal environment (fluid)* that all cells live in and to which they are continuously exposed. The regulation and balance of this internal pH within the human body is a *"vital"* function; thus it is imperative that this environment is kept constant and is controlled with *exactness* and *precision*. Just like a fish immersed in the appropriate type of water, fresh vs. salt, your cells are living in a specific biological fluid environment, bathing in an extra-cellular fluid environment (outside the cell), as well as maintaining an intra-cellular fluid environment (inside the cell). The most important fluid every cell in our body will be "bathed" in is blood. Through the vascular system's most intricate and delicate complexity, blood and the contents it carries will be distributed throughout the body, eventually reaching every cell. So crucial is the regulation of the pH balance of our human bloodstream that it is recognized by *all* medical physiology textbooks as one of the most important biochemical balances in *all* of human body chemistry. *All biochemical and electrical reactions and energetics of cellular life are under pH control.* Therefore, your body is working every second to balance this delicate ratio of acidity to alkalinity (basicity).

In order to understand the physiological process at work that is utilized to maintain this acid-alkaline balance, one needs to know exactly what "pH" refers to. The term "pH" is a measure of the acidity or alkalinity (basicity) of a solution (in chemistry it is defined as the potential hydrogen concentration). We can measure and assign a number from one to fourteen to describe whether a solution is acidic or alkaline (basic). Solutions with a pH less than seven are said to be acidic. Solutions with a pH greater than seven are said to be alkaline or basic. Solutions with a pH of seven are said to be neutral. Our blood system maintains a *narrow* pH range for optimum physiological functioning: between 7.34 to 7.45. From these numbers we can see that *human blood is slightly alkaline or* basic. Human blood must inherently be able to continuously and accurately regulate this critically narrow pH range, thereby maintaining its alkalinity for optimal cellular/organ system functioning.

Let's now examine how this balance is maintained. The main physiological system at work creating pH balance is unique and known as the "buffering" system utilized by our blood. Remember that our blood is alkaline. If the environment moves toward increased levels of acidity, even to ever so slight a degree, the buffering system (bicarbonate system) will neutralize the acidity and restore the pH back to the balanced alkaline state. This reaction to shift the environment from acidity (lower pH) back to alkalinity (higher pH) by the buffering system of the blood takes only a *fraction of a second*. This enables a rapid shift back to alkalinity and minimizes over all drastic pH changes. The slightest shift, again a pH decrease towards acidity, has profound, destructive effects on human physiology. For if in fact the pH of our blood shifts too much towards acidity, we will die! Because every cell metabolically produces acidic wastes, this buffering capacity of our blood system will constantly be at work striving to maintain pH stability, thus bringing about optimal balance (*Homeostasis*). So, as the Bible says, *"the life is in the blood."*

It should now be clearly evident that this internal terrain will impact every cell and biological function within the body. As described, any minute deviation from this alkalinity is a "sign" that *Homeostasis* is being disrupted and that danger to our health is manifesting. Symptoms that arise, indicating dis-ease, are the "signals" of eminent danger to our health and wellbeing. A host of disturbing biochemical changes and malfunctions ensue when the pH balance is even slightly distorted toward acidity. These include:

1. Regulation of what enters and exits the cell

2. Structure and function of *all* biochemical molecular structures, including life-sustaining enzymes

3. How efficiently and productively molecular components are utilized

4. The utilization and vital assimilation of carbohydrates, fats, proteins, vitamins, and minerals

5. Major to subtle metabolic reaction disruptions (including energy depletion)

6. Cell to cell communications (both systemic and local)

7. The ability to transport gases is severely compromised, including the delivery of oxygen, ("molecule of life"), to cells and toxic carbon dioxide gas away from cells

8. Nervous system signal transmissions are impaired

9. Organ systems become crucially compromised (***Immune system***, brain, liver, heart, etc.)

10. Increased susceptibility to pathogenic attack by viruses and bacteria which can even mutate and change shape, becoming increasingly infectious and more difficult to fend off

11. Irregular growth and division of cells (e.g. cancerous cells)

It is quite interesting to note at this point that Hippocrates, centuries ago, said, "Let food be thy medicine, and medicine be thy food." We can even extend this further to include the type of fluids we hydrate our body with as well. When foods are metabolically broken down, the respective components are either life-supporting or life-destroying. ***All foods, and what we drink, collectively shape the internal terrain of the body.*** If one examines the history of medicine and the theory of disease, the well-noted Louis Pasteur's contributions of the germ theory are highlighted with great emphasis, praise, and accolades. There were, though, other scientists who laid down profound discoveries of how diseases manifest within the human body. One of them was Claude Bernard who spoke about the internal terrain of the body and how it relates to illness and disease. His work indicated that it is the "milieu" or the environment that is all-important to the manifestation of diseases. Microbes, as he maintained, do change and evolve, but how they do so is a direct result of the environment or terrain to which they are exposed. Disease within the body will develop and manifest, depending upon the state of this internal biological terrain. At the core of this biological terrain is pH. Yet, the main focus of medicine relentlessly centered on Pasteur's germ theory, which honed into germs and disregarded the effects of the biological terrain in which they were flourishing. It is said that on his deathbed, Louis Pasteur acknowledged that Bernard was correct, the microbe is nothing, the terrain is everything. This was a complete turnaround from his proposed original germ theory, demonstrating that there were flaws all along in his theory. By this time, medicine had latched on tightly to the germ theory, solely focusing on the "germ," irrespective of the terrain in which it was thriving.

There are other examples of profound discoveries in human physiology and medicine which, after being documented in biological texts and receiving prestigious awards, have been quickly brushed under the table by modern allopathic medicine. Doctor Otto Warburg was one of the greatest contributors to the field of cell biology (he also mentored other great scientists who made exceptional contributions). He is responsible for the discovery of "key" enzymes involved in cellular respiration (the collective biochemical reactions from which cells derive their energy in the form of ATP). He investigated the metabolism and respiration of cells, including cancer cells, and in 1931 was awarded the Nobel Prize in physiology/medicine for his discovery of the "nature and mode of action of the respiratory enzyme." He was nominated for another Nobel Prize years later. His extraordinary contributions continued to dominate within the field of cell biology. He also became known for his work in the area of the pathogenesis of cancer cells. In 1924 Warburg postulated that cancer cells mainly generate energy (ATP) by *non-oxidative (low oxygen)* breakdown of glucose, a process known as glycolysis. This is in contrast to "healthy" cells that generate energy mainly from the *oxidative (high oxygen)* breakdown of pyruvate, the end-product of glycolysis (this process is aerobic respiration occurring in the mitochondrial organelle). Malignant cells that grow rapidly typically have glycolytic rates *(low oxygen pathway)* that are up to 200 times higher than those of their normal tissues of origin. This phenomenon is referred to as the Warburg effect. Warburg articulated his findings in a paper entitled "The Prime Cause and Prevention of Cancer" which he presented in the lecture at the meeting of Nobel Laureates on June 30, 1966. In his own words, "the prime cause of cancer is the replacement of the respiration of oxygen in normal body cells by a fermentation of sugar."

Warburg's work also tied into the proper balance of the internal terrain and pH. He wrote about oxygen's relationship to the pH of cancer cell's internal environment. Warburg reported that cancer cells maintain and thrive in a lower pH (acidic) due to the fact that they utilize fermentation as their major metabolic pathway. This pathway produces lactic acid and elevated CO_2. This demonstrated the correlation between pH and oxygen levels and the type of cells that will thrive, depending upon the conditions. A higher pH (alkaline) means a higher concentration of oxygen; healthy cells will thrive in this environment. A lower pH (acidic) means lower concentrations of oxygen; cancer cells will thrive in this environment. Utterly convinced of the accuracy of his conclusions, Warburg expressed dismay at the continual discovery of cancer agents and cancer viruses which he expected to hinder the necessary simple *preventive* measures.

It is known that the process of cellular metabolism , the oxidation (breakdown) of nutrients to produce energy for cells to function, creates residue waste products that must be eliminated by the body. They are toxic and acidic. If we are not *completely* and *efficiently* eliminating these waste products produced by the trillions of cells of our body, they will get stored somewhere within our body. No matter how pure the food we consume, our cells still produce acidic waste products that must be discarded regularly. Any accumulation, buildup, and storage of these cellular acidic waste products will contribute to cellular dysfunction and tremendous early aging.

A fascinating experiment was carried out by a famous French physiologist, Alexia Carrell, whereby he kept a chicken heart alive for about twenty-eight years. Carrell, incubated a chicken egg, removed the heart of the developing chick and sectioned it into pieces, each one consisting of numerous cells. These pieces were transferred into a saline solution containing minerals in the same proportion as the chicken blood. By changing this solution everyday, he was able to keep the chick's heart alive for about twenty-eight years. When he stopped changing the solution, the chick's heart cells died. Why were the cells able to survive for so long? By changing out the fluid every day, he was discarding the cellular waste products (acidic) produced every day and keeping the extracellular fluids (the terrain) mineralized (alkaline) and constant.

In the early 1930's, Weston A. Price, a dentist from Cleveland, began a series of investigations that were quite unique. His goal was to discover the factors responsible for good dental health. For over ten years, he traveled extensively to isolated parts of the world to study the health of populations untouched by western civilization. Dr. Price's studies revealed that dental caries and deformed dental arches, resulting in crowded, crooked teeth, were the result of nutritional deficiencies. This finding was contrary to the explanation that inherited genetic defects were the cause. Wherever he traveled throughout these areas, he found that the people with proper nutrition had straight teeth that were free from decay. He also found these people were resistant to diseases and had healthy, good physiques. What he observed was that these qualities were typical of native groups on their traditional diets, diets that were rich in essential nutrients. Dr. Price analyzed these foods consumed by these isolated people and found that they provided at least four times the water soluble vitamins, calcium and other minerals, and at least ten times the fat-soluble vitamins which act as catalysts to mineral absorption and protein utilization compared to the American diet of his day. Interestingly, the fat-soluble vitamins came from a variety of foods we have shunned as unhealthy. The photographs of these isolated people with their beautiful teeth and bone structures, fine physiques, ease of reproduction, emotional stability and freedom from debilitating degenerative ills stood out markedly in contrast to civilized modern lifestyles where people subsist on devitalized, processed, and packaged foods, refined sugars, white flour, pasteurized milk, low fat foods, and abundant convenience foods filled with conditioners, additives, and preservatives (many of them to extend shelf life). Dr. Price's discoveries and conclusions were written up and presented in his classic volume, *Nutrition and Physical Degeneration*. It documents striking photographs of healthy primitive people and illustrates, in an unforgettable way, the abundant physical degeneration that results when human groups abandon not only nourishing traditional diets, but nutrient dense, enzyme rich, mineral balanced, non-toxic wholesome foods.

Dr. Price's work clearly illuminates how the healthy expression of human physiological function, form, and unique constitution are dependent upon the fulfillment of a variety of nutrient/ mineral-rich foods. These foods, as they are broken down within the body, provide the daily requirements for cellular function and create the integral and balanced internal terrain for every human cell to thrive in or malfunction in if disproportionate in their components.

It is absolutely regrettable that modern medicine has completely turned its back on some of these greatest scientific discoveries in human physiology. This brilliant work, elucidating ways in which the body operates physiologically and perpetually keeps *Homeostasis* at bay (a necessity for human biological life to continue and thrive in an optimally well way), has been abandoned and irresponsibly ignored. Medicine refuses to acknowledge these discoveries which medicine itself originally embraced (briefly though), published, and awarded the highest recognition. How can modern medicine blatantly ignore these inherent physiological working principles while attempting to provide a "so-called health solution?" The answer is, they simply cannot! They have ignored these principles or pay attention to a few and claim to be healing us. What should have been logically and responsibly developing within western medicine are, for example, doctors specializing in internal pH analysis and its restoration through physiologically compatible avenues such as diet, herbs, homeopathy, etc. It is medicine's duty to embrace and implement ALL of these physiological discoveries and work in harmony with them if they are to attempt to heal. At present it is up to us to embrace, support, and seek options that are aligned with these inherent physiological working principles in order to resurrect our health and wellbeing.

Now, the logical question arises: what types of foods contain bio-available nutrients that your cells have evolved to recognize and will contribute to the maintenance of the internal pH terrain? Until that time when we can design a genetically engineered cell that can derive bio-molecular components to function from synthetically processed and chemically modified foods, human cells will require pure, wholesome, unrefined, non-synthetic, unprocessed, unadulterated foods, *real* foods. There is a glut of modified, manipulated, processed, and preservative-laden foods on the market today. These are "toxic" and "deadly" to human microscopic cells. They poison the internal terrain. They are void of essential biochemical nutrients. The constituents of these foods are incompatible with human physiological functioning. We should not manipulate foods at the high cost of impairing *Homeostasis* and the body's working physiological intelligence. Thus, common sense tells us *real* foods should be eaten and a wide variety of them. We should be eternally grateful that nature has provided us with copious varieties of wholesome foods and ones that naturally provide antioxidant benefits. The molecular components of these foods have evolved to be recognized and efficiently utilized by cells. The variety of foods nature provides us with should be rotated on a regular basis, incorporating fresh, seasonal varieties as much as one can. We must also consume the foods known for their antioxidant properties. The majority of these foods should also be alkaline producing in nature (approximately 80%) and a lesser amount of acid forming in nature (20%). Foods considered alkaline contain minerals such as sodium, potassium, magnesium, calcium, and iron. This means that these foods leave an alkaline ash residue following cellular metabolism, thus complementing and supporting the inherent alkalinity of our body's physiology (mentioned earlier). Foods considered acidic contain minerals such as sulfur, phosphorus, chlorine, and iodine. This means that these foods leave an acidic ash residue following cellular metabolism. Thus, in order to avoid an over-acidic internal terrain, these foods should comprise a smaller amount of your diet. The chemically modified, manipulated, processed, preservative-laden foods all create abundant acidity in addition to the harmful properties mentioned already and should be avoided if possible. If one does not focus on shifting away from these acidic foods, one is heading for disastrous health outcomes. A degenerative domino effect, systemic in nature, will be set in motion, resulting in a detrimental condition known as Acidosis. The majority of one's health challenges relate to Acidosis and once again, not surprising at all, western medicine is oblivious to this simple shift that creates inordinate needless suffering for millions and millions of people.

If you nourish your body with foods in these proportions (80/20) and *real* foods that are high in nutritional density and inherent vibrational energy, your cells will naturally be able to run efficiently as they have evolved to do. Synergy and coordination between the trillions of cells inherently will be at work. A cell that is operating efficiently, synergistically and in coordination with other cells is a healthy cell. Healthy cells thrive in an alkaline pH environment. Healthy cells can make all necessary adjustments for *Homeostasis* to be maintained. These cells at some point in time will divide and create more healthy cells (mentioned above), provided you choose the *wholesome, real* foods nature has provided us with (and a higher percentage of the alkaline forming foods).

As cells carry out their work, breaking down structures and reforming new ones, various acidic waste products are produced which **must be** eliminated. Healthy cells and a diet compatible with their optimal functioning will not be over-burdened by excessive amounts of these acidic wastes and will adequately efficiently, and appropriately eliminate them. This will ensure an internal terrain that is balanced, slightly alkaline, and that resonates with the body's inherent *Homeostatic terrain* to support over all health. This is another reason why good **quality** foods and the ratios mentioned above are essential.

If we nourish our bodies with poor quality, over processed, synthetic, chemical laden, genetically engineered, manipulated foods which are toxic, devoid of essential life-sustaining nutrients, and all overly acidic, our precious cells will struggle. They will fight for their lives to obtain constituents needed to support their structure and function. These remarkable entities, the microscopic center of human life, *your life*, will be struggling and fighting just to maintain their existence, let alone fulfill their physiological purpose. Imbalances on all levels will begin setting in, e.g. the pH will shift toward acidity, impairing cellular functioning, and depriving them of the abundant energy necessary to thrive. In order for *Homeostasis* to be maintained, an internal battle will ensue, resulting in a cascade of uneven biochemical events. Like Robin Hood, taking from the rich and giving to the poor, robust, nutrient plentiful cells and tissues will be robbed of essential components by the poor, depleted, imbalanced cells fighting to maintain their existence. For example, minerals and other nutrients will be leached from tissues and cells of one organ system so cells of another organ system can maintain their existence. Disruption of the *Homeostatic* steady state will result, creating total chaos within the body. The result will be disastrous. Your amazing microscopic cells will immediately suffer. In time, if we fail to properly nourish them they will become dysfunctional, massively stressed, will run out of energy, prematurely age, and will eventually shut down or die. Is it surprising then that we experience abundant illness, dis-ease, and needless suffering? Common sense tells us no!

Thus, it is again imperative that we understand **why we eat** and how *precious* good food is. Yes, we want to enjoy food and we should, but we can also develop a keener awareness as to what foods would best support the physiological demands of our body. Also, we can begin fostering an immense appreciation for the thousands of unique varieties of foods nature provides us with, and the beautiful ways in which they develop into their edible forms. Now, with *gratitude and appreciation* of foods, and orienting yourself with this mindset, you can make wiser choices with greater ease. These choices will inherently begin encompassing and taking into account the nourishment of particular organ systems, providing premium fuel for cellular demands through foods which are more compatible with our sensitive alkaline pH. Wellness within will begin blooming.

Water

Water is the "liquid of life." The foundation of the human body is water. We develop within water and water is *vital* for *optimal* physiological functioning throughout life. A fetus developing in a mother's womb mirrors our evolutionary path from early life forms originating in the sea to a human being. The amniotic fluid surrounding the fetus cradles life. This fluid is mostly water. We develop within this fluid. Trillions of cells divide and differentiate within nine months, the **majority** of each cell being composed of water. Water is the foundational liquid and "universal solvent" which carries nutrients to the fetus and carries toxic wastes away. At the appropriate time, we will emerge from the sea of life. From early human life, beginning with fetal development, through older age, water remains the "liquid of life." The majority of our human body is composed of water, approximately 80-90%.

Throughout life, the body is **critically** dependent on adequate amounts of "pure, health- promoting water" to function properly. A human body can survive for weeks without food, but when water is absent for even a few days, the body will suffer dire consequences (dehydration). Water is vital to **all** biological processes in the body. The trillions of human cells within you are dependent upon water as are the magnificent molecular constituents and biochemical reactions. *All* biochemical molecules involved in human physiological structures and functions are dependent on water. Every biological process within our living system occurs in water. For example, the movement of muscle tissue is possible because it is mostly comprised of water. The instructions that muscles receive are via nerve impulses transmitted through water. Your eyes move freely because of their lubricant consisting mainly of water.

The presence of adequate amounts of proper water and its molecular orientation directs all bio-molecules, once synthesized, to take their unique, respective shape and become bio-chemically active. This includes the most versatile molecules: enzymes (the catalysts of virtually every biochemical reaction); antibodies and surface cell structures of the immune system that recognize a wealth of foreign structures; and key signaling and receptor molecules throughout the body. None of these are biologically able to precisely perform their duties in the absence of adequate amounts and right type of water. Without their proper structure and shape, these bio-molecules are ineffective in their intrinsic functions.

The majority of human blood and lymph fluid is comprised of water. Water is **crucial** for healthy blood and lymph flow, the former often referred to as the *"river of life."* It is a crucial factor in the blood's ability to efficiently transport precious oxygen and nutrients to cells and carry toxic, acidic wastes, including carbon dioxide, away from cells to be discharged. Water is essential for efficient enzyme activity, immune function, metabolism, lubrication of joints, brain function, and proper digestion, including the activation of intestinal bacterial flora, just to mention a few. Eighty percent or greater of all health challenges relate to dysfunctional digestion and poor intestinal health. Water keeps various tissues moist, ensuring protection against the invasion of bacteria and viruses; thus it is a natural contributor to our defense system. Water is essential for proper osmotic conditions and pressure (osmosis is the movement of water/solvent across a semi-permeable membrane), leading to proper water and salt balance inside/outside cells. These parameters are essential for optimum health. Water is the medium through which cellular signals travel (nervous system transmitting signals from brain, etc.). Water, the "universal solvent," is vital for the distribution and delivery of **ALL** nutrients to their appropriate destinations; it is also vital for toxic, deadly acidic wastes to be discharged and eliminated from the body. The kidneys are a most spectacular display of physiological brilliance in this regard, continuously keeping a delicate *homeostatic* balance between water, minerals, and various nutrients, while efficiently eliminating excesses including toxic, acidic waste products from the body. Water is the perfect means of energy transfer within biological systems because of its capacity to hold so much energy. Water turnover, the amount of water entering/exiting the cell, contributes to energy production. Most people are not familiar with this. Thus, if we are slightly dehydrated, our energy levels are inherently affected as well, energy goes down.

If the volume of "pure, health-promoting water" is below the body's requirements and is inadequately distributed, a host of serious, chronic, debilitating life-threatening health challenges ensue. The result is disastrous and leads to cellular dysfunction. Cellular energy diminishes, malnourishment of cells will arise, biochemical components will begin malfunctioning (as mentioned above) and cellular communication will be disrupted. Acid wastes and toxins will accumulate due to the inability to be excreted properly and efficiently (for example, gout). Internal acid waste and toxin build-up will lead to further disturbances, such as decreasing the pH of body fluids which will affect all cells, shifting them from a healthy alkaline pH to an acidic pH (the stomach is acidic when hydrochloric acid is present to digest food). In addition to the multitude of malfunctions that will result, this accumulation of acid wastes and toxins will eventually profoundly affect the over all health of cells as well, causing serious, irreversible damage to molecular, cellular components, including all protein structures (distortion in structures, denaturing of enzymes, dysfunction of immune structures, etc., as mentioned) and the most important molecule, DNA. The brilliant harmony of cellular interactions and organ system functioning is now impaired. Moreover, how can a cell with all of these compromises duplicate/replicate and copy themselves with the new cells being any healthier than the parent cell? They cannot! This duplication of cells, which occurs frequently throughout the body, will give rise to progeny that are less than optimal in their functioning. Simply stated, adequate amounts of "pure, health-promoting water" are *vital* to the extraordinary delicate balance, *homeostasis,* within the body. We, along with the majority of doctors, believe that one should drink water only when we are thirsty..... the body says otherwise. Studies have shown that by the time we are actually thirsty, we are already dehydrated at the cellular level. Thus, we should continuously be hydrating with water throughout the day.

It should now be clearly evident that water is the foundation of human physiological functioning. **Within our living system, every biological process takes place in water.** Providing your body with adequate amounts of "pure, health-promoting water" *directly* affects human health, wellness, and longevity. Paying attention to not only the amount of water we drink, but the **type** of water we drink is *essential.* This will have a *greater positive* influence on our health than anything else. The supply of proper water to the body can itself bring about the most fantastic healing and reversal of health imbalances within the body plus helping prevent numerous health challenges and premature aging.

Not all water, though, supports the delicate yet rigorous requirements the body demands. Tap water these days most certainly does not meet these requirements. It contains high amounts of chlorine and numerous other harmful chemicals and toxins, all of which pollute and oxidize the water. These additives create *free radicals* which result in detrimental, degenerative effects on cellular health. *Free radicals* (unstable/highly reactive structures) wreak havoc on all levels of cellular function as they strip away electrons (negative charge) from other atoms and molecules. In the process of the free radical's attempt to become stable (stealing

away a negative charge from another atom/molecule) they create additional instability of biochemical structures around them,
now leaving these structures unstable. This result then causes
more damage to other structures, a domino effect is set in motion which becomes difficult to halt. It is true these additives kill
off micro-organisms that can harm the body, however, the human body does suffer. Chlorine itself, added to water, destroys
the symbiotic life-giving relationship that proper water offers to
the friendly flora inhabiting the intestinal tract, thus killing off
the majority of these friendly organisms. Tap water becomes acidic by the treatment processes and contaminants dissolved in it,
counteracting the body's natural, healthy internal alkaline environment. The acidity created by these additives are counter-acted
with the addition of more caustic *chemicals* after treatment (Lye)
to neutralize the acidity so that it will not corrode the pipes it trav-
els through. More attention is paid to the effects on the "pipes"
rather than to the human body! Oxidation of the water creates
not only destructive *free radicals*, but imbalances and distortions
in the molecular shape of the water molecule aggregates, causing high numbers of individual water molecules, H_2O, to cluster
together. These very large clusters are not able to efficiently penetrate the cellular membrane to provide adequate cellular hydration and remove deadly toxic, acidic wastes. You recognize that
super full feeling in the stomach after drinking this water.

Our cultural obsession with bottled water, along with the numerous types, variations, and wondrous claims, including all of
the designer and sports waters, is far from meeting the requirements of cellular physiology either. The plastics containing it and
the length of time the water is in contact with the plastic containers creates toxic solutions. It is a fact that bottled waters may sit
on a palate in the sun (at the distribution location, warehouses,

or the market) for days to months before we consume it. These waters are also high in *free radicals* and acidic. Even though the manufacturers claim these waters are alkaline and electrolyte enhanced, vitamin infused, etc. these waters measure as acidic as caustic sodas! They are devoid of essential utilizable alkaline minerals (ionized)! The irony is that the manufacturers begin with reverse osmosis water, water that is considered "dead water" due to the lack of vital minerals. Yes, this water is "filtered," however, the essential minerals are also filtered out and what remains is not suitable for our body's physiological demands. The attempt is made to restore this water to some type of healthier state by adding back various components like minerals; however, again, they are not in a utilizable form (ionized) for the body. Another factor which most people are unaware of is that bottled waters are treated with various compounds to prevent the growth of harmful bacteria after it is capped/sealed (Chlorine, Fluorine compounds, etc.). If only a few bacteria are present after the capping of these containers, they can exponentially multiply and create a sea of bacteria. Thus, these types of waters are degenerating cellular health and counteract the natural alkaline environment the body requires (similar to tap water). These waters have not only become toxic, acidic, and oxidized, but they also contain individual water molecules, H_2O, which have associated into clusters that are far too large for proper cellular membrane penetration and toxic acidic waste removal. In fact, these clusters are often larger than the aggregates formed from tap water!

What is the upshot of all of this? Our precious water, the simple *"liquid of life,"* has been manipulated to a degree resulting in the degradation of our health upon consumption. The alarming part is that we spend billions of dollars on bottled waters and drinking tons of it. We are also consuming large amounts of tap water which has been treated with various harmful chemicals (mentioned previously) that directly affect our health. The properties of these waters are enemies to our overall health and wellbeing, quite the opposite of the properties true nature provides and of water that is found in pristine sites in the world. Too many people are pumping lots of water into their bodies, but what kind of water is it? You may be attempting, with good intentions, to support your body's hydration demands by drinking good amounts of water; however, you may not be aware of all these chemical alterations which affect water's properties, structure and capable function and how that impacts health. All health professionals should know these basic biochemical principles surrounding water. Considering this is the *"liquid of life,"* it is truly perplexing that doctors, following their medical training, are not even capable of instructing us about what kind of water we should be drinking and whether the amount we are consuming is adequate to support the daily biological demands of the human body to secure an optimum level of health. Since the majority of the human body is comprised of water, this should be the ultimate place to begin resurrecting health, drinking health promoting water and enough of it.

What water meets the daily complex physiological hydration demands? What water maximizes nutrient absorption and utilization while at the same time meets the removal demands of harmful acidic cellular wastes? What water interacts in a biologically compatible manner with biological molecular structures? What water contributes to creating a suitable intra/extra cellular environment to bring about the most efficient communication, functioning and optimum wellness within the body? Is such water available? Yes it is. Abundant research shows that tap water can be restored to a natural health promoting state. This water is called *Ionized* water, electrolyzed water, or often reduced water. Research demonstrates that it does in fact fulfill the biological needs our body demands. In nature, water constantly undergoes *ionization*. *Ionization* of water, in simple terms, is the splitting apart of the water molecule into two components. This process is also referred to as self-ionization, auto ionization, or auto dissociation. This is what we call a reversible reaction, whereby the two components are also autonomously coming together again to reform a water molecule after their dissociation. Thus, water splits apart and reforms continuously. Without getting too much into complex chemistry, this process, ionization, creates what is called 'reduced' water. What this means is that an abundance of anti-oxidant properties are generated naturally by this process. Remember, that harmful free-radicals are unstable structures that "steal" negative charge away from other molecules, thereby leaving those structures unstable. This is called oxidation. Anti-oxidants contain high amounts of negative charges, thus they can donate them to neutralize and block the harmful effects of free-radicals. So, ionized/electrolyzed/reduced water naturally contains high amounts of negative charge which is available to neutralize the harmful effects of free-radicals. Thus, this water is a natural, beneficial anti-oxidant! Studies show that this type of water is much higher in anti-oxidant properties than foods that rate as good anti-oxidants! In addition, when the healthy minerals—Sodium, potassium, magnesium, calcium—are present in the water when ionized, the individual water molecules are unable to aggregate into large clusters as mentioned previously. These properties translate into immediate absorption and utilization in addition to the other positive qualities mentioned.

The beauty of this whole process is due to the simple biological principle of electron (negative charge) transfer. Simply put, *all* biochemical reactions involve the *transfer* of electrons (some molecules gain electrons, some lose electrons). Remember, when a water molecule, H_2O, is ionized, it splits into two parts (negative and positive ions). Not only is the water dissociating, but the resulting charged ions are now additionally able to further ionize minerals if present in the water, creating a host of 'active' biochemical reactions. These types of cascade reactions are constantly occurring in the body naturally. If these "active" biochemical reactions eventually cease, critical impairment of cellular functions can result, even leading to death. Unfortunately, with all the treatments and manipulations of water, including bottled water (mentioned above), this vital process is inhibited; thus, (again) all the **critical** health promoting properties water should be providing our human physiology are absent.

Ionized water can be efficiently re-created through electrical means for our consumption. The Japanese have been using the *highest* quality ionized water for decades (Kangen[R]) to abundantly restore a host of health challenges, prevent numerous debilitating illnesses, combat premature aging, and maintain over all wellness. It should be noted that the Japanese are consistently ranked the healthiest and longest-lived culture. The health benefits of consuming this water are so dramatic that it is currently in use in hospitals throughout Japan and has been for over 40 years. It is now an adopted practice in their overall socialized medicine structure. Additionally, The Japanese Association of Preventive Medicine for Adult Diseases endorses its consumption since they find it so effective. What is it about this water that makes it biocompatible with our physiology and comprehensively fulfills the body's hydration needs and the removal demands of deadly acidic, cellular wastes? There are several basic, restorative properties that emerge upon ionization, truly returning source water to its viable health promoting origin just like water found in nature and pristine places around the world (sadly decreasing in number).

One of the restorative properties of this water is a higher alkalinity. This is due to higher quantities of *essential* alkaline, ionized minerals and a higher amount of hydroxide ions. Alkaline water inherently has a higher oxygen content due to the high hydroxide ion content and lower hydrogen ion content. The source water flowing into the ionizer contains a mixture of minerals, both alkaline and acidic. A good ionizer (eg. the ones used in Japan which are 'medical devices') filters out harmful substances, but leave the healthy minerals in the water (sodium, potassium, magnesium, calcium) as well to be ionized. Upon the completion of ionization, two types of water are created, alkaline and acidic: positive, ionized minerals, which are alkaline minerals, namely magnesium, calcium, sodium, and potassium, are separated from negatively charged minerals, which are acid minerals, namely chlorine, phosphorus, and sulfur. These ionized alkaline minerals along with the hydroxide ions raise the pH of the water. Thus, a healthier alkaline water emerges for consumption. By the way, the acidic components mentioned above are separated during the ionization process and discharged out of an ionizer. The pH of this water is low, acidic. It turns out, the ionizers (Japanese medical device units which we can actually purchase) can create an extreme acidic water which is safe and efficacious for certain health challenges (killing bacteria/viruses plus more) and for sanitizing/ disinfecting uses! This acidic water has been approved in Japan for disinfecting in various settings (Hospitals, food prep areas, schools, plus more).

Back to the alkaline water. This water affords the body essential beneficial properties. One of them is that it imparts an *increased* buffering capacity to assist in the neutralization of excess acidity within the body. As mentioned earlier, our blood system has evolved with a most exquisite alkaline buffering system (chiefly bicarbonate) to assist in the maintenance of its pH (7.35-7.45, slightly alkaline). This buffering system is **vital** to human health and can be easily and quickly used up, the result of which is chronic dis-ease, abundant health challenges, and premature aging. Oh yes, let's not forget death! If the body gets too acidic it will shut down. Drinking this alkaline water extends the buffering capacity, thereby increasing the amount of acidity that can be neutralized, thus reducing the overload on the bicarbonate buffering system. This, in turn, diminishes and eliminates the devastating effects over-acidity will cause (remember, acidosis impairs cellular/muscular function and can be deadly). Tremendous health benefits automatically result from an increased capacity to buffer (neutralize) an over-acidic internal terrain. Research has also shown, these alkaline minerals contribute to the stabilization of small water cluster structures which are essential to proper hydration and our over all health.

The health promoting benefits of this ionized water increase even more due to the tremendously high anti-oxidant properties of the water, another most important property. The anti-oxidant properties of a substance are measured by its oxidation-reduction potential (ORP). This measurement, the ORP, will be either a positive or negative number. Positive numbers reflect oxidation, while negative numbers reflect anti-oxidation properties. Water with a high negative ORP (-ORP) is of particular value. It is a *superb* anti-oxidant. This translates into a most abundant and effective ability to neutralize free radicals! Remember, all chemical reactions involve a transfer of electrons. Some atoms or molecules are described as being "electron poor" and will steal or strip electrons away from another atom or molecule, thereby oxidizing that entity. These are highly unstable molecules that are *oxidizing* agents due to their *deficiency in electrons*. They must strip electrons away from one entity, leaving that entity unstable and now in need of stealing electrons away from another entity to fulfill its stability. Molecular structures of normal, healthy tissues all around will be subject to attack by these predators. This goes on and on creating a most devastating chain reaction. All these electron deficient entities are collectively called 'free radicals.' Free radicals are among the most damaging molecules within the body. They degenerate, damage, and deteriorate physiological components within the body and result in disease and aging. Oxygen free radicals are the most potent destroyers and are known to contribute to a wide variety of harmful, life-threatening health conditions, as well as a host of less threatening yet debilitating, chronic health conditions.

Some atoms or molecules are described as "electron rich" and will donate electrons to another atom or molecule. They are termed *reducing* agents due to their *abundance of electrons* to donate. Another way to state this is that they have a high reduction power. They are able to donate electrons to the entities that are lacking electrons or have been stripped away. They carry the potential to neutralize and stabilize free radicals, including oxygen free radicals and their destructive domino affects; therefore, they are referred to as anti-oxidants. Ionized water, with its *high reduction power* (negative ORP), has abundant electrons to donate, affording it *supreme anti-oxidant properties*. It is naturally capable of neutralizing and stabilizing the abundant and constant damaging effects of copious free radicals, especially oxygen free radicals, within the body that cause the horrific degradation of our precious health and premature aging. This water's anti-oxidant properties rise high above foods that are categorized as anti-oxidants (these are also electron-rich donors and alkaline) and we can consume a lot more of it more easily than foods. Since the majority of the human body is composed of water, and we need to consume an abundance of it, what a simple health fortifying solution it provides. What a blessed *"gift"* this *"liquid of life"* is to our human physiology.

Lastly, ionization *naturally* shifts the molecular clustering of source water back to how it is found in nature, restoring another **key** property. This molecular structuring includes the number of water molecules, H_2O, and how they are organized into clusters. Ionization (electrolyzation) reduces the size of water clusters. Each individual water molecule is bent shaped (like an upside down "V") with unpaired electrons on the oxygen atom. Chemists describe this as a 'polar' molecule—an uneven distribution of electrons (one side is more negative, the other side more positive in charge). These water molecules find stability by joining hands with neighboring water molecules through hydrogen bonds between them, creating **small** clusters. One of the most natural, stable, and extraordinary health promoting groupings is known to be the hexagonal geometry and it has been shown that various alkaline minerals are responsible for contributing to their structural stability by strengthening the bonding between them (structure-making ions), as well as increasing their number. The properties of this structured clustering now impart numerous powerful effects including an ability to efficiently and rapidly hydrate, efficiently discharge deadly toxic acidic wastes, generate copious amounts of energy, and stabilize DNA and protein structures.

The addition of caustic chemicals and/or the removal of all good alkaline minerals, in tap or bottled water (mentioned above), create destructive distortions in water molecules. These distortions lead to water clustering in very large, unorganized aggregates. These large aggregates (highly unstructured) contain anywhere from ten to thirty or more individual water molecules joined together, a far greater number than the small hexagonal geometry of ionized water, and will be incapable of fulfilling the multitude of essential biological functions required by water. This leads to compromising health issues. In contrast, ionization, effectively reduces the size of the water clusters. The alkaline minerals (mentioned above) are considered structure-making ions as they strengthen the bonding between these grouped water molecules, thus creating *small*, hexagonal structures. Additionally as mentioned, an increased number of these small, stable clusters results as well.

It has been determined, and research shows, that human beings and other biological organisms prefer this small clustered, organized geometric structure—it will *profoundly* affect over all health by directly and indirectly supporting biological functioning. A demonstration of this can be seen if we consider, for example, blood plasma and its components. The two major components are water and protein, approximately 90% water, 7% protein. As you can see, water comprises the majority of this fluid, thus the aforementioned properties (amount, size cluster, geometry of water) will impact every cell and molecular structure within the blood as well as every cell and molecular structure it eventually comes in contact with upon circulation throughout the body. Another fascinating aspect surrounding these properties is that various layers or states of water surround protein structures. It has been shown that one protein molecule has an average of 70,000 water molecules immediately surrounding it. These water molecules participate in valuable ways in structurally supporting the numerous folds and bends of the large protein molecule, thereby facilitating its function and protecting it from outside disturbances (remember enzymes which are crucial to biological reactions are proteins).

Protein molecules are not the only molecules to benefit from such water's positive relationship. The genetic *"molecule of life,"* DNA, is also surrounded by structured water molecules. It has been shown that normal DNA which has a helical shape is surrounded by highly structured water of this nature (properties mentioned above). This water is much less mobile than the water surrounding abnormal DNA. This tightly held and highly structured water surrounding normal DNA, acts to stabilize its unique helical structure and forms a layer of protection from all sorts of outside influences which could cause malfunction, distortions, free radical attack, and mutations that create abundant serious physiological problems (this includes the generation of abnormal, cancerous cells). Numerous additional molecular structures throughout the body, whether simple ions or larger molecules, positively interface with this type of structured water (Molecular Water Environment Theory). What a *beautiful* symbiosis and exhibition of the extraordinary intricate workings of biology are seen with the **right type of water.**

The excitement surrounding ionized water continues as its health promoting benefits are amplified even further. Remember, water is the medium in which all bodily functions take place. It has clearly been shown that this structured water improves cell water turnover. Smaller hexagonal units of water, as opposed to larger, unorganized conglomerates of water, are able to penetrate cells more rapidly and can efficiently assist nutrient absorption, waste removal, and cellular metabolism. This type of water also prevents the loss of essential cellular minerals, balancing the external to internal cellular ratio so vital for proper cellular functioning. The greater amount of total water movement (rate of cell water turnover) *directly* impacts metabolic efficiency—the higher the turnover, the higher the metabolic efficiency. Both cell water turnover and metabolic efficiency have been shown to be important markers for over all health, including weight balance, longevity, and aging. Our energy levels are also tied in with these processes. An additional fascinating finding is that overweight individuals have a reduced amount of total body water (up to 20% less than a normal individual). Since overweight individuals have a reduced metabolic rate and this correlates with total body water and cell water turnover, increasing the consumption of ionized, structured water provides an inherently natural and simple resolution for weight balance.

One of the biggest challenges for any biological organism (one that will also facilitate weight loss) is the removal of toxic wastes from its system. Every metabolic cellular function produces acid wastes which, if not removed efficiently, can lead to acidification which then destroys the health of tissues and organs. This over-acidification has been correlated with both disease and aging. If an organism can eliminate these wastes more efficiently, its over all health, vitality, and life expectancy will be enhanced.

Hexagonally structured water also has a huge capacity to store energy. Therefore, it has a larger caloric capacity and greater ability to perform "work." This energy is immediately available for release when utilized by living organisms, making it the obvious biological choice. Since it has this capacity to hold so much energy, it is also the perfect means of energy transfer within biological systems—it is energetically more powerful!

You must now agree that paying attention to the *type* of water we drink will unquestionably impact *every* level of physiological functioning, keeping the body working at its peak performance. By drinking the right type of water, we can easily renew, restore, and maintain the delicate balance required of our precious internal "sea of life." Divine wellness will manifest and vibrantly grow, naturally flowing and circulating throughout our brilliant bodies.

Words and Thoughts

The trillions of cells making up our bodies are a microscopic, collective, massive, vibrational, energetic entity. In addition to their basic physiological structure and functions, they contain vibrational energetics (or vibrational current) which play a key role in over all health and wellness. Cellular structures are formed from a variety of different atoms and the way in which they are arranged into larger molecules. This in turn dictates the respective functions found either within the cell or on the surface. These molecules can also be released from the cell and circulate throughout the body where they now can partake in numerous additional reactions. Each of these atoms and molecules carry their own intrinsic vibrational energy. *Homeostasis* is dependent upon harmoniously resonating molecular and cellular energies and interactions among them, which autonomously lead to proper internal/external cellular function, cell to cell communication and the abundant, finely orchestrated physiological interactions occurring every second within the body. An electrically charged flow or current generated from the vibrational energies circulates throughout the body as cells carry out their work, and the array of the biochemical constituents are interacting perpetually and energetically in a harmonious fashion.

At the foundation of these energetics lies the simple composition of the atom, a basic unit of all matter, and its interaction with other atoms to create larger molecules. Every atom has a nuclear core containing protons (positively charged) and neutrons (neutral). Surrounding this core, the nucleus, are energy levels where electrons (negatively charged) are found occupying distinct spatial areas, known as orbitals. These subatomic particles impart an inherent amount of energy within the atom. A variety of atoms or the same atoms can unite through the interaction of electrons, either through the sharing of electron pairs or the donation of electrons from one atom to another, thus creating a bond between them. The variety of combinations that can be arranged make it possible for the vast number of cellular components to form and carry out their functions. Atoms bond together to make up the abundant molecules found within the cell, on the surface of our cells, or released from cells to interact with other distant cells elsewhere in the body. The bonds connecting atoms carry an inherent amount of potential energy as well as vibrational and rotational energy, the collective energies of which create the electrical current flowing throughout the body.

How does this relate to the words and thoughts we daily choose and their impact on your over all health and wellness? Words and thoughts carry energy as well. Words and thoughts are like atoms and molecules, carrying intrinsic energy, depending upon connotation. Letters are like atoms strung together, creating words that are just like molecules. Words are then chosen by us and used in our thoughts. The energy of words which create our thoughts can either constructively or destructively interact with our cellular energy, thus creating a positive or negative influence on cellular health. Words or thoughts encompassing such things as resentment, hate, ill will, fear, anxiety, doubt, anger, struggle, or deprivation tear down the health of the cells of our body and systemically poison our blood. They destructively interact with the energies of cells. They block the vital energetic flow from cell to cell and they drain cells of their intrinsic vital energy. Over time, the abundant, coherent biochemical reactions are disrupted and distorted and the nervous system is energetically shocked. The resulting outcome is dis-ease and illness of various forms. The energies of these types of words and thoughts are also highly acidic. Highly acidic words and thoughts produce high acidity in the blood (shifting the healthy alkaline pH as mentioned earlier). This, in turn, affects every cell and organ throughout the body, another major contributor to the destruction of health and wellness.

Since your words and your thoughts carry associated energies, they too impart an electrical flow through your body. This electrical energy, when flowing, will instantly interact with the electrical energy flow generated by the molecular constituents mentioned above. Again, this energy constructively or destructively resonates with it, thus having a positive or negative impact, even a complete chemical and/or electrical shift within your body's physiology, depending upon what type of words or thoughts are chosen. The continual choice of words and thoughts with destructively resonating energies and acidic words and thoughts will begin shifting the body's internal terrain (mainly pH). The over all balanced energetics of the internal terrain will become distorted and the environment will move towards a more acidic condition, thus severely impairing all cellular function over time. This impaired cellular function will, in turn, affect the functioning of our organ systems. Different organ systems will be affected at varying rates. As the energetics continue to be disrupted and the pH shift begins, the destruction will gain great momentum, quickly translating into numerous health challenges.

We do, though, have complete command over what words we choose to use and the thoughts we create with them. Since energy is neither created nor destroyed, only transformed, you can begin transforming the choice of destructive words and thoughts you use into energetically constructive ones, thereby restoring the over all energetics of the body. These words and thoughts will also begin shifting the internal terrain, compatibly contributing and restoring the inherent alkaline internal terrain of the body. How can we become our own effortless master of transformation to immediately restore and redirect this vital energetic flow? By mastering the *"Art of Mental Transmutation."* The word "transmute" means to change from one nature, form or substance into another. This principle is usually employed to designate the ancient art of transmutation of metals, particularly simple base metals into gold. Among the numerous *secret* branches of knowledge possessed by the ancient Hermetists was that known as *mental transmutation*, wherein one could change or transform mental thought, states, forms, and conditions into others. Thus, you can see that practicing *mental transmutation* is practicing the *"Art of Mental Chemistry."* Your words and thoughts, just like metals and elements, may be transmuted from state to state, degree to degree, condition to condition, pole to pole, and most importantly, *vibration to vibration.* As this is achieved, one will experience profound positive transformations in all areas of one's life, most notably health.

Masterfully utilizing mental transmutation produces words and thoughts that are energetically constructive and alkaline in a process that is immediately available. Mental transmutation means producing loving, kind, encouraging, happy, joyous, positive, grateful words and thoughts. Through these energetically constructive new words and thoughts, you will now have a wealth of transformed electrical energy at your fingertips to direct like a magical wand over your body. As a result, an energetically harmonious, balanced, and healthy vibrational internal environment will transpire with the choice of these types of words and thoughts. Additionally, any over-acidity will begin shifting back to the *homeostatic* alkaline state.

It is known that words of **love** and **gratitude** possess the highest positive vibrational energy. Again, you may be asking how this can assist you with your health? The answer is: through the non-resistant, secret principle of transmutation. Again, energy is neither created nor destroyed, only transformed. The "Art of Mental Chemistry," as mentioned above, will transform the electrical internal environment and the energy of cells. Transmute your words and thoughts into the highest energetics of love, gratitude, appreciation, and joy. Words and thoughts of this nature will electrically reprogram cellular energy. These words and thoughts will also alkalize your blood, thus creating a balanced *"river of life."* Begin with the incorporation of **love**, for divine love running through you will dissolve all seeming obstacles. It will immediately make your path clear, easy and successful. Divine health and wellness will flow to you at an unobstructed, endless rate. **Gratitude** also carries these high resonating energies and alkalinity. Continue building up a magnificent energetic, alkaline portfolio of words and thoughts of such nature. In a very short period of time you will achieve the masterful mental transmutation of words and thoughts and will reach vibrant new physiological energetics and balanced internal pH terrain. *Now watch with absolute amazement as you experience the most magnificent, magical shifts within your body, shifts toward increased, unstoppable health and wellness.*

I highly recommend enlisting others you can team up and work with to master this art. Not only will you have support, but you will also have others who can point out to you words or thoughts that are so habitually destructive and that you are not consciously aware of using in the beginning. You can also make a game out of the process if working with others. Choose people who are genuinely as interested as you are in mastering this art and transforming their vibrational world. If there is any hesitancy or criticism along the way from the people you chose or people who express interest, let go of them immediately. They will polarize you in the opposite direction away from the mastery you are seeking. If no others are interested in joining you, team up with vibrationally compatible books (use the authors as your mentors) or other information you can consistently read to keep yourself on track and keep yourself in motion toward mastery of this art. While developing your masterful skills, you need to absorb and bathe yourself in the highest degree of like energies to the ones you aspire to resonate with.

Once you learn how to consistently transform and transmute the old patterned words and thoughts, thereby changing both your internal and external vibrations, your conditions will shift in wonderful ways. You will even notice in time that others all around you will be affected in a positive way as well; they will want to seek out this alchemic process you are following in order to shift their internal and external vibrational conditions.

Nature

Nature Offers "Free" Prescriptions for Health

It is crucial that we take time to understand and fully appreciate nature along with all of the inherent healing benefits it has to offer us. Our health and well-being are "critically" dependent upon the abundant healing relationships between nature and our health. Nature provides us with *"free"* prescriptions to restore, rebalance, and maintain our health and well-being; however, we need to be aware of what nature's benefits have to offer us in order to take advantage of them. There are an extensive number of extraordinary processes and healing gifts nature presents to us every second of every day, yet the majority of us are unaware of them and/or unaware of how to utilize them. As our society has become more urbanized—working in enclosed buildings, on computers/phones for long hours, seeing mainly concrete surroundings, i.e. concrete mania, etc.— our connection with nature has diminished and the impact upon our health and well-being has been *greatly* compromised.

When we take the time to understand, appreciate, and indulge in these relationships with nature and the numerous health benefits we can profit from, a new world will magically open up for us! You will be on your way to *Mastering Wellness*.

We are **living** entities and truly blessed to exist within the **living** world of **nature**. We are partners with *nature*. Our relationship with *nature* is a symbiotic one—we have a mutually beneficial and interdependent relationship with *nature*. We would not exist if all that nature provides us with did not exist. At the same time we help *nature* flourish. There is a delightful, harmonic balance that exists between *nature* and ourselves. Are you aware of this symbiotic world?

One of the most profoundly beautiful symbiotic relationships that demonstrates the above, exists between *Cellular Respiration* and *Photosynthesis*. Humans and animals carry out the process of *Cellular Respiration*. This process involves Oxygen which is necessary for the production of energy molecules critical for life. We breathe in Oxygen from the environment, it combines with various molecular components (from the breakdown of our foods) inside the cell and water, and produces utilizable energy in the form of the molecule ATP (Adenosine Tri-phosphate). A byproduct of *Cellular Respiration* is Carbon Dioxide (CO_2) which is released from the body through breathing (exhaling). It's a fact that without the production of this energy molecule, ATP from *Cellular Respiration*, we would not exist!

The process of *Photosynthesis* is carried out by plants. Plants take in the Carbon Dioxide from the environment (remember, we exhale Carbon Dioxide through breathing every second), combine it with other molecular components inside their cells, and produce sugars and energy molecules necessary for their growth and life. The byproduct of *Photosynthesis* is Oxygen....... just what we need for our *Cellular Respiration* and life. The by-product, Carbon Dioxide, of *Cellular Respiration* is what humans and animals release into the environment and plants absorb for their utilization of life. The plants, in turn, release Oxygen into the environment for our lives. This is a magnificent and beautiful display of symbiosis.

Since there are so many magnificent aspects of nature's benefits for the human body, it would be too much to mention all of them here; however, the following descriptions and insights are a start to enable you to begin your *Mastering Wellness* journey. Utilize these examples to educate and inspire yourself to begin orienting a Wellness mindset around them. This will blossom over time, not only into fostering a life-long appreciation for nature, but the pursuit of establishing a healthy relationship with nature to support your health and well-being.

You know that refreshed feeling after being by the ocean or the awe of the fire red sunset over the ocean; the breath-taking feeling when we see a magnificent view; the sheer astonishment when we see flowers with extraordinary vibrant colors or delight in their wondrous scents; the calm feeling around green trees, mountains, or plants; the peace and purification being around a creek, babbling brook or fountain or the exhilaration upon hearing roaring rapids or waterfalls; the smiles when we hear beautiful birds chirping or owls hooing; or the enchantment as the wind blows over us or we see the dancing and flickering of leaves and branches of trees and plants. But why do we feel this way?

We, humans, have five basic senses: Sight; smell; hearing; taste, and touch. They all play an important role in human physiology. Our body utilizes them every second of every day of life. They all work together in various ways without our even thinking about it. Our brain receives signals/stimuli from each of these senses, interpreting and utilizing the information for our body accordingly. All of the senses play a role in our overall health and well-being. As open land has been transformed into concrete plains, confined buildings consume our society, long hours in enclosed vehicles stifle us, and long hours on computer/phone devices deplete us. Thus, our interaction with nature and engaging these senses is lacking. In addition to this, there is the spectacular open 'space' of nature into which our inner spirit is craving to expand and interact. It doesn't take much to satisfy the body and its nature 'fix.' For example, most people notice immediately when they go to the beach, that they feel 'different' in a good way.

Another example of a *free* health prescription from nature is the beautiful *symbiotic* relationship between the *sun* and the *human body's production of Vitamin D*. Vitamin D is essential for health. It plays a role in bone health, cardiovascular health, neuromuscular system health, diabetes, prostate health and more. Its best known role is keeping bones healthy by increasing the intestinal absorption of calcium. Without enough Vitamin D, the body can only absorb 10 - 15% dietary calcium, but 30-40% absorption is the norm when Vitamin D reserves are normal. The fascinating thing is that only minuscule amounts are required for health; however, it must be available for utilization by the body. Although Vitamin D is firmly enshrined as one of the four fat-soluble vitamins, it technically is not a vitamin. Vitamins are defined as organic compounds (carbon-containing) that must be obtained from dietary sources because they cannot be synthesized by the body's tissues. Vitamin D, however, is manufactured by the human body. Vitamin D is absent from all natural foods except fish and egg yolks, but even when obtained through these foods, it must first be transformed by the body into other forms before it can be utilized. Vitamin D is not just one substance, but many. The first step of Vitamin D production occurs in the skin from a universally present form of cholesterol, 7-dehydrocholesterol. **Sunlight is the key component** necessary for transformations that need to occur before the final version of Vitamin D is active. **Sunlight's ultraviolet B (UVB) energy** converts this precursor to Vitamin D$_3$. Thus the *Sun's energy* turns a chemical component in your skin into Vitamin D$_3$. This, in turn, is carried to your liver and then your kidneys to transform it into active Vitamin D. Along the route, this form picks up extra oxygen and hydrogen and eventually the final active version emerges, *Calcitriol*, which we name Vitamin D.

A question most people ask is: Can we just take a supplement? Yes, you can take a supplement if necessary, however, as you can see from this example, we have evolved to obtain this compound, Vitamin D, utilizing the energy of the sun. This is the most effective way to generate the utilizable component we need for optimum health. Living in these modern times we have diminished an essential symbiotic relationship with nature, the sun, and Vitamin D production. Many people, including our most valuable future, our children, are greatly suffering from a lack of Vitamin D. As mentioned previously, we are obsessed/addicted to phones and high demands have been placed on us for computer use. We spend an enormous time indoors (long work hours, etc.) and kids have a bare minimum of physical activity in school and have been consumed by the video game craze, additionally adding to a reduction in physical activity and time spent outdoors. Concrete is replacing open land. All of these factors add barriers between us and nature.

Ah, how alive and exuberant we feel when we take our shoes off and walk in the sand, put our feet in the ocean water or cool flowing stream bed, or put our bare feet in the grass. Why is this?

The earth upon which we live has a 'frequency' or 'heartbeat' called the Schumann Resonance, approximately 7.83 hertz. The Schumann resonances, named after their discoverer, drive the harmonizing pulse for life in our world. This rhythm has played a major role in governing the evolution of life. We all march to the cadence of the earth's drums, so to speak. This planetary heartbeat sets the tempo for health and well-being, meaning this resonance and number it turns out are extremely important for human health and well being. Remember, we are *living* entities with a frequency and rhythm as well. The human body and earth both have electrical charges or fields. Thus the earth can influence our body's human charge. You have heard that when we stand on the ground (barefoot), our body is grounded. Simply put, in a "tuned" system of oscillators (the human body and earth), when one oscillator begins vibrating, the other oscillator will eventually begin vibrating at the same frequency. This process is referred to as "entrainment" or "kindling." Fascinatingly, this Schumann resonance falls within the range of human brain waves, precisely the middle where the alpha brainwave and theta brain wave ranges meet. In other words, we vibrate at the same frequency as the earth does and we use this to survive and thrive. This is why scientists attribute being out in nature to be so enlivening and healing for humans.

We have evolved in synchronicity with the earth's frequency/ heartbeat. Without the earth's resonance and our direct contact to it (eg. being barefoot), our health can become compromised. NASA scientists have known this for quite some time. Astronauts in early space missions became surprisingly weak and ill when they ventured into space and left the earth's resonance behind. In order to compensate for this, a vibrational device, resonating at Schumann's frequency would be attached to the space ships. Thus, by providing the astronauts with Schumann's resonance, they were able to synchronize their frequency to that of the earth they left behind. Why is this important? Our environment has become increasingly polluted with electromagnetic fields (EMF's) which wreak havoc on the human body (cell phones, cell phone towers, computers, etc.). In addition, as society has evolved we spend an abundant amount of time indoors (for work, etc.) with artificial elements, are surrounded by seas of concrete, and we have shoes on that prevent us from physiologically connecting with the earth. Since early human times, we as a species were barefoot and connected to nature (i.e. hunting, gathering, farming, even sleeping outdoors).

Documented stories from the Native American Indians describe how they have also known how important it is to be in contact with the earth. When Indians were sent off to Oklahoma (Sioux, Navajo, Apache, etc.) and relocated to reservations, the kids attended the 'white man's schools,' wearing their clothes and cutting their hair. When the kids came home from school, their mother's would say "take your shoes off; if you don't, you know you will get sick."

Research shows that numerous health challenges are attributed to the formation of "free radicals." These are unstable, positively charged atoms that have lost one or more electrons (negative charge). They hunt, like predators, to steal negative charge from other atoms to create stability again. This process in turn damages cells causing illness, inflammation, premature aging, and more. Chronic inflammation has been implicated in a host of common health issues, such as rheumatoid arthritis, arthritis, multiple sclerosis, heart disease, Cancers, diabetes, plus more. Antioxidants are negative ions. These negative ions have extra negatively charged electrons. Negative ions, therefore, can neutralize those destructive positive ions, the free radicals. It turns out, that negative ions are abundant in nature. This is why we feel so good for example, around waterfalls, the ocean, green trees and plants. Negative ions create positive vibes. Research is showing that negative ions, upon reaching the bloodstream can produce biochemical reactions that increase levels of the mood chemical 'serotonin.' This helps alleviate depression, relieve stress, and boost daytime energy. Negative ions also clear the air of airborne allergens such as pollen, mold spores, bacteria, and viruses. Again, the mechanism is that they attach to these positively charged particles in large numbers to neutralize harmful effects.

Thus, here is another free prescription from nature — negative ions!

As we can see from these examples, nature has abundant healing benefits for us to utilize free prescriptions for health and well-being. This wondrous world of nature is available right this instant for you to seize and begin your *Mastering Wellness* journey. No matter how much time you devote — several minutes to several hours to days or weeks — immerse yourself in some aspect of nature. Play, frolic, take a moment to stop and smell the roses. Appreciate the colors, scents, sounds, and tastes of this magical world. Take a break at work, take your shoes off outside, and put your feet on some grass. Sit under a tree for a few minutes. Observe the flowers and the delightful scents. Take note of all the varieties of plants and trees around you. Create time everyday for a little dose of nature, it will do your body good. No matter how or what you do, the action will become infectious. You will begin to 'crave' and appreciate nature around you. Lead the way and inspire others on your journey. In no time your body will smile back with positive outcomes while you are taking delight in nature.

"People who know nothing about nature are, of course, neurotic because they are not adapted to reality."

"Nature is not matter only, she is also spirit."

—Carl Jung

Taking the First Steps for Mastering Your Wellness

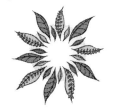

Begin your journey by *acknowledging* your decision to make changes. Be proud of yourself for making the decision and grateful for the timing of your decision. No "should of's would of's, or could of's." Create the most *loving appreciation* of your body, its extraordinary innate intelligence and physiological brilliance, for it is the trillions of cells within your body that will transform your efforts into the wellness desired. Be gentle, kind, and loving to yourself along the way. Give yourself loving permission to *enjoy* the endeavor; take whatever time you need; be as creative as you need; experiment and learn whatever you need along the way. There are no mistakes and no absolute right or wrong decisions. Don't let any opposing forces, including fears, doubts, past experiences, etc., yours or anyone else's, halt the journey you set in motion. Create your own internal voice of continual, loving *encouragement,* no matter what stage you are at. *Transmute all relative discouragement into unwavering faith and determination*

to create and own your divine optimum wellness. Commit to only taking this path and know that with this commitment will come divine universal support. Expect abundant wellness favors along the way—people wanting to assist you, new avenues of support to connect with, pertinent information related to your state of health, new practitioners with enlightened compassion, and new modalities. Expect magical miracles at any point in time. Within your heart you know how you want to feel and look (or if you are assisting a child or family member, how they want to feel). Within each man is a *super-conscious* mind—God mind—infinite intelligence—wherein lies the realm of perfect ideas. Plato spoke of "the perfect pattern," the "Divine Design." There is a Divine Design of wellness for each of us. See this perfect picture, expect it can be achieved, believe, and begin creating it. The masterpiece will be the completely transformed, ***vibrantly healthy and well "YOU."***

All obstacles NOW vanish on my path. Every door flies open, gates are lifted, and I confidently sail into my kingdom of wellness, under grace and in the perfect way for me.

An artist who is beginning a new project is like a curious detective. The Artist may test a new color or a combination of colors to see how they blend, test various brushes or tools, test different techniques, or the medium he/she desires to work with. The artist may begin on a small scale or jump in on a large scale. Become your own curious, artistic wellness detective. Take a simple, small step or a bold, big step and begin building around it. Choose one of the four foundational areas above to begin, again creating small or large but consistent shifts. For example, evaluate some of your thoughts and choice of words. If they are negative, defeating, or destructive in over all vibrational energy, or acidic in substance, transmute them. Choose new ones. Begin diluting the old ones and as you dilute them, begin infusing your vocabulary with more energetically supportive, alkalizing, positive, constructive vibrational words. Use these to formulate new thoughts and build a whole new thought pattern. As you do this, your body will inherently create a whole new internal wellness pattern from these transformations. You will be amazed at how efficient you become in the process of transmutation—quickly shifting your choice of old words and defeating thoughts into new ones. I am confident you will have fun as well. You will begin noticing a completely new physiological energy within you. You will feel energetically bright, light, and alive, and your internal terrain will begin restoring itself autonomously. Health will begin growing within as you resonate in this new place. Watch as new doors fly open for you everywhere and effortlessly lead you where on your journey you need to go next.

If you choose to begin in the area of foods, apply the same principles. Two of the greatest challenges many people face when it comes to dietary changes are fear and intimidation. Often these fears surround change and letting go of the old with the uncertainty of the new. You cannot be split between fear and/or doubt and faith. Trust and faith must permeate every step of your journey. If a tree is to be transplanted from one place to another, its roots first will be dug up and freed from the surrounding ground. They will be completely exposed. A nice, new environment will be prepared, paying particular attention to the needs of the tree's roots. We all know the roots are the life giving structures. The tree, with its roots, will then be placed in this new area, making sure the roots are firmly and happily attended to for survival in this new growth environment. The roots will not choose two paths for the tree's health and growth, some roots switching and growing above the ground due to doubts, the other growing deeper into the ground with the knowledge of trust and faith. All roots will follow the latter growth pattern—trust and faith. They will resume their inherent growth pattern, extending themselves deeper into the ground, securing the tree into the soil and continuing to spread themselves out, maximizing their ability to absorb nutrients and water, fortifying the tree's growth and securing life.

Intimidation often surfaces as a feeling of tremendous pressure to change everything overnight. It surfaces and brings immense burden, literally paralyzing us from taking any action. Remember, you are the artistic wellness director of your health. If you need to, begin with small steps, like an artist's fine strokes. Whether you choose to take small or big steps is not important, but consistency and continual action are.

With an objective eye, observe and evaluate with *kindness* your diet and food choices that you regularly make. Take the opportunity to investigate ingredients. Choose a food you regularly eat that is not as healthy for you and find a healthier replacement. If you do not like the choice you first make, you are free to try again and again and again..... Slowly begin diluting the less healthy food from your diet while introducing the healthier ones. Remember, you are *free* to creatively experiment and enjoy the process. You may be eating foods that contain high amounts of sugar, salt, unhealthy fats, deadly and toxic artificial sweeteners, or chemical preservatives/additives. Begin choosing foods with more wholesome ingredients. Of course, the more pure, the greater the physiological benefits. And, YES, abundant alternate choices are out there, ones that you will enjoy and your body much prefers! Remember, you are *free* to creatively experiment, while enjoying the process. Any way you choose to make these shifts is all right. As you incorporate these changes, with amazement you will notice, in a short period of time, your body literally speaking out to you and saying it likes these changes. Your body's preferences will autonomously move away from the hold of the old and be redirected to the new and beautiful bold choices you are making. Again, give yourself permission to slowly acclimate to these changes and know that they will continue to flourish with greater ease. Your body will continue speaking to you, letting you know it is feeling better by the absence of debilitating symptoms and the emergence of a host of health improvements including: increased energy; improved digestion; weight balance; improvement in sleep; mental clarity; enhanced mood; fewer colds/flu's; decreased headaches; less joint pain/stiffness, plus much more. Your immune system will be forever abundantly grateful for the changes—refined sugars and chemical preservatives/additives all *dramatically* reduce immune system function and *deadly, toxic* artificial sweeteners are just that, "**toxic and deadly**" to all cellular health. A more even physiological balance will emanate as well—a sign that *homeostasis* is now being restored. Let the momentum continue and assist you in building upon these accomplishments. Confidence in your ability as well as confidence in your body's abilities will strengthen. Keep in motion the infusing of new foods into your diet, one in place of the other, one more healthful than another. Look to the vast array of natural, biologically compatible wholesome foods nature has gifted to us. There are endless tasty choices for everyone. Rotate different foods and explore varying seasonal foods as well as rainbows of colors of different fruits and vegetables. Increase alkaline foods, try incorporating some raw foods, even juicing. You will discover delightful new favorites you wished you had known about all along. Then watch as wellness blossoms, the masterpiece emerging.

Remember, you are the master artist. Experiment, have fun, and give yourself permission to be infinitely creative. As this philosophy continues in motion, remember Newton's first law: Every object in a state of uniform motion will remain in that state of motion unless an external force acts on it. Don't let yourself or anyone else be the "external force to stop your motion. You can keep wellness in motion by being aware of and keeping opposing, destructive forces away. Just as transmutation of your words and thoughts will become second nature, so too will the transmutation of foods and dietary choices. Your body will be absolutely in love with the changes you make, taking off by what it well knows how to do—restore *homeostatic* balance. By fueling it with superior quality foods, water, and thoughts, its innate intelligence will be your master guide.

You may decide to begin with water, changing the *type* of water and increasing the amount you drink. I strongly encourage you to shift to ionized water, incorporating it into your *daily* living routine. You will be watering your body with the most blessed gift of a lifetime.

Coffee, tea, soda, juice, milk, etc. are **not** replacement beverages for water. Health promoting water must **reign supremely** at the **top** of the beverage list. Many beverages should be eliminated altogether. Choose one beverage you drink that you know you consume too much of. Now with that artistic masterfulness, find a tasty alternate. You can choose and re-choose as many times as you like. When you come upon the improved choice, begin diluting the less healthy one and infusing the new one into your daily routine. Again, you may be able to make an immediate shift or you may need a more gradual approach. Either way is all right. Sadly, many unhealthy beverages are addicting and can pose a challenge for some to eliminate (e.g. caustic sodas). It is a fact that as you increase the consumption of "pure, health promoting" water, your craving for unhealthful beverages will decrease. Slowly, your body will adjust to the change and begin feeling better. Of course, the sooner you can eliminate unhealthful beverages altogether, the better! In no time at all, your body will feel so much better it will not want the same amount of sugary, degenerating, caustic, acidic beverages. If you try drinking more, your body will intelligently tell you "**no**!" Consider this: it takes 32 glasses of 'strong' alkaline water (pH of approximately 9.5) to neutralize one glass of man-made cola with its pH of 2.5! Another example is if one drinks a lot of coffee. Your body will appreciate gradually reducing the higher amount consumed. Use the dilution method by reducing the ratio of coffee to water. This will facilitate the reduction, in a gradual manner, in the number of full-strength cups you consume daily (even consuming half-decaffeinated at the same time). Your body will begin to re-acclimate to the reduced amount of caffeine, and in time you can continue working towards completely eliminating the caffeine or reducing it to a more minimal level. Incorporating ionized, alkaline, micro-clustered water into your wellness regimen will assist your body even further, neutralizing harmful, acidic effects these beverages impose and opening up a wealth of new channels for the body's physiological intelligence to reach. When a beverage, such as coffee, is made with this water, not only will you need less coffee to make a cup but you will automatically neutralize the over-powering, degenerating acidity of the coffee. It is a win-win situation all around and once again a blessed "*gift*" to your body.

The outcome of these implemented changes will again result in your body letting you know that it no longer likes these types of liquids. Once again, your body will guide you and let you know it is feeling better over all. How? Your body's inner intelligence will speak to you as mentioned above with changing food choices. These signs are telling you it likes what you are doing, so keep it up. That is the fun part! What will the body continue to do with this momentum? It will achieve even more health in a shorter period of time and with greater ease.

No matter where you begin or what you choose to shift first, *all* roads will lead to wellness. The masterpiece is being created. Begin in one of these areas, let the momentum build, keep constructing upon it, mix and match, be creative, explore, experiment, learn, and most importantly, have fun with it! Magic will happen.

As your body begins to feel better physically, your emotional state will elevate, leading to a much greater sense of motivation. The momentum you set in motion will pick up pace, over-riding any initial resistance and will continue leading you down your wellness path. A clearer plan will take shape with regard to the action you need to take, such as changing doctors, seeking a more holistic practitioner, complementing with other modalities, or pursuing a combination of disciplines. You may not even need any previous options you thought were necessary! This new, more vibrant, energetic state you are in will also attract a host of events and circumstances that will manifest in support of creating wellness. I recognize and acknowledge that there may be some legitimate barriers; however, I cannot condone excuses. Everyone can make an investment at some level, for without health there is no life. The path towards wellness will save not only needless suffering and abundant money, it will **save your LIFE!**

Resurrecting Your Health

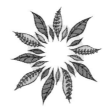

The time has come. "Now" is the time for creating divine wellness for you, your family, or a loved one. We are all deserving of this. Needless suffering can be lifted. The chronic dis-eases we have learned to accept can be abolished, as the majority of them are completely preventable. Each and every one of us is a precious soul, a most miraculous biological organism, with unique God-given talents. Choose to take charge of your health and wellness now without delay; become a master and lead the way. Set into motion a wellness journey today and watch the momentum grow. Transforming your health will inspire others to begin their journey. This will keep you motivated and continuously re-inspired. Transforming your health will contribute to paving the road for others to transform their options. As we actively create health and wellness ourselves, western medicine and society at large will be forced to follow along. In fact, the energy and momentum of wellness will be so *brilliant* that everyone will want to follow the path. The abundant wavelengths of wellness will now be powerful enough to constructively transform morbid suffering and the current state of health crisis into joyful celebration for all. We will be the Resurrection of Health movement.

My Goal for You

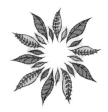

I hope you are inspired and joyfully illuminated with refreshing insights. May your divine new wellness plan (or your family's or a loved one) now easily unfold right before you with grace and in perfect ways.

Say to yourself:
Now is the appointed time; today is the day of my
amazing good fortune. Miracle after miracle and wonder
after wonder will ensue. I now look with absolute amazement
at the health and wellness masterpiece that has
divinely manifested itself before me.

I have faith in you and believe in you. You must adopt unwavering faith yourself, believe in and embrace the extraordinary intelligence of your body and your abilities to master success. Expect the best results. I know optimum wellness is now a part of your life. I see your masterpiece, the **healthy, vibrant and well "YOU."**

All my love and blessings go out to you for a joyous and successful **Resurrection of Your Health.**

My Resurrecting Health Favorites

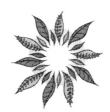

Mastering Wellness 'Buddies'

The following are just some of my favorites:

Chia seeds - I love this amazing tiny food. Don't let the size fool you! They contain all the *essential* amino acids and are loaded with omega-3 fatty acids. The Tarahumara (Raramuri) people of Mexico are renowned for their long distance running ability. They are known as the "100 milers." They run anywhere from 100-300 miles, eating *only* Chia seeds and drinking water along the way!! Wow!

Ionized, Alkaline Water - *A gift of life*. My body LOVES it! Your body will love it. My favorite is the Japanese units that simply hook up to your faucet (Enagic). These units are in over 300 Japanese Hospitals. The water is an integral part of their socialized medicine program and has been for decades. Additionally, it is endorsed by the Japanese Association of Preventive Medicine and the Association of Anti-aging.

I turn my faucet on and "Voila," this water is made fresh in seconds.....NO plastic involved!

And remember..... your body consists mostly of water!

Homeopathy - It works! It is safe for any age! Choose the right single remedy, a combination of remedies, and a solid experienced company, and apply modern, proper dosing....feel the effects. Homeopathy has been around since the late 18th century and in spite of its rich source of disputes, you can find the science backing it along with clinical positive effects. It is amusing that we forget that some of the most effective western prescription medicines come from natural plant sources originally.

Barefoot-ing - I love being barefoot when I can. Stretching my feet out, engaging my whole foot, including my toes. You are feeling the earth, grass, sand, or any of natures surfaces and 'grounding' as well. It helps you stay healthy, promotes healing, and is calming yet invigorating. **Ahh!**

Xero Shoes - Based on *natural movement* (barefoot-inspired principles), these shoes are amazing. No matter what activity you engage in, they have a shoe for you. Natural movement means happy feet; happy feet mean happy body; happy body means a happy and healthy mind..... you get it :)

Vibram FiveFingers - Dancing and prancing with a huge smile on my face, that is what happens when I run in these shoes :). Also a barefoot principle shoe. One will automatically adjust to proper barefoot techniques and enjoy whatever activity you choose.

Water - In addition to what I like to drink (mentioned above).... I love water! I love the sound of flowing water, swimming and wading in it, dipping just my feet in it, splashing it, and watching reflections. It has such an invigorating vibrational as well as calming effect. Water is the *"liquid of life" for the mind, spirit, and body.*

Nature - I *love* being out in nature. It offers our *"free"* prescriptions for health. It is magical and wondrous. I love observing and being around trees, looking at the individual differences in their overall structures—leaves, trunks, colors, locations. They each have an authenticity just like us. I love sitting by or underneath them.....listening to leaves dance, watching the light impart its beauty upon the subject, or absorbing the negative ions. Flowers are a favorite of mine also. A divine work of nature. I call them *smiles from the universe.* With their exquisite, multitude of colors and shapes and their delicate or bold fragrances, they smile at us boldly and bravely no matter what their size. Birds are angels in flight, soaring, coursing, exhibiting the utmost freedom.... Take joy watching them in flight or of course observing them anywhere they are. These are just some of the pleasures nature offers.

As Carl Jung said, "people who know nothing about nature are, of course, neurotic because they are not adapted to reality."

Shaklee - All nutritional supplements are NOT the same! The quality of the raw materials, especially where plants are grown and the content of the soil, how they are formulated (combination of vitamins, minerals, herbs, nutrients need to be balanced), and consistency in the product make-up are *key* to their effectiveness over and over again. Experience in the science/research of products are of the utmost importance as well. I want to know who is making what I consume for my body. These products are the choice of Olympic Athletes and Astronauts whose bodies' demand the highest level of physiological nutrition.

Growing/Harvesting Fruits, Vegetables, and Herbs - Whether it is a small basil plant, a bunch of carrots, an established big orange tree, or a large garden one can truly appreciate our foods and nature when we plant, watch the growth, and harvest any category of edible food. Sheer amazement and gratitude comes through me when I plant something and watch it grow from seedling to maturity. It is mind-boggling to know that a tiny seed when planted, fed, and watered will eventually take form into a mature complex organism. It is a gift to oneself to not only eat the food, but to know why we are eating foods and where they come from.

Stevia - This plant is native to Brazil and Paraguay. Often called *"sweet leaf"* or *"sweet herb,"* Stevia rebaudiana has been used *safely* for health for *centuries* by the Guarani peoples of South America. This plant has many health benefits including pancreatic health and regulating blood sugar. It turns out that one of the properties of the plant is that the leaves taste sweet! The leaf of the Stevia plant is known to be 200-300 times as sweet as sugar due to steviol glycosides (mainly, stevioside and rebaudioside). That's right, sweeter than sugar and it is a plant! I love it in my teas and other beverages when I want a *little sweetness* added. Many people have expressed to me over the years that they do not like the taste.....if you have tried it and that is the case, fear not, try other brands and forms (liquid, powder, etc.). When grown and prepared properly, it adds a most pleasant sweetness and aids in regulating blood sugar. What a *"sweet"* food it is!

Music - Music is and has been for centuries the *healing voice of the world*. It has been and is an integral part of healing and communication within numerous cultures throughout the world. The vast numbers of sounds and combinations of them we can create with numerous instruments is astounding. These varying sounds all carry unique vibrations. It is known and research has shown that music has a tremendous positive effect on human physiology and animals as well. You may like to listen to music or you may want to learn to play an instrument. I love listening to opera when running, the strength and freedom of the voices flow through my body, strengthening my legs and core, and put rhythm in my stride. I also play the Djembe drum. This instrument along with other African drums are rooted in healing, communication, and entertainment. So choose your music—sounds, instruments, tempo—let the the music flow.

Bison - I am not a big meat eater, but when I do want meat I *love* bison! It is America's original red meat. Nutritionally it is hard to beat. It has higher iron than beef; higher vitamin B-12 than chicken; lower fat than beef or chicken; and contains a high ratio of healthy fatty acids like omega-3. It is very nutritionally satisfying and one feels the difference. Bison have natural patterns of grazing, patch grazing, which contribute to a healthy environment and ecosystem.

Appendix

Kangen® Water by Enagic International

Pioneering, Revolutionary Technology

Kangen®water, the sole trademark of Enagic International, is pure, health- promoting, *ionized (high anti-oxidant), alkaline, micro-clustered* water produced by Enagic International's pioneering and innovative water technology. For over four decades, Japanese based Enagic International, has been the *leading specialized manufacturer* of alkaline water ionizers. By integrating the foremost scientific research and superior Japanese craftsmanship with nature's most vital resource in "life," Enagic has pioneered the way in producing this *precious water* on a daily basis right from your faucet's tap water.

Enagic International supplies hundreds of hospitals and thousands of restaurants with industrial-sized alkaline ionizers. These water machines are also used in millions of homes worldwide to transform tap water into pure, ionized (high anti-oxidant) alkaline, micro-clustered drinking water. Enagic's systems not only produce health promoting Kangen^R water for consumption, but also produce acidic waters for various uses. The acclaimed, strong acidic water has been approved and is used throughout Japanese hospitals, restaurants (including food product disinfection), and schools for **non-toxic** disinfecting and sanitizing. Additionally, it is used as a safe, non-toxic pesticide.

The individual water ionizing units produce water of varying pH's that can be used on a daily basis with confidence to benefit and improve health and beauty, complement cooking (used in Japan for the preparation of foods, drawing out delicate flavors and textures which both the chef and consumer appreciate), and non-toxically clean, disinfect and sanitize.

In 1965, the Japanese Health and Welfare Agency approved ionized water devices using electrolysis as *medical equipment*. The electrolysis machines Enagic International manufactures in Japan and sells throughout the world are *licensed medical devices* and have been granted a license number by the Japanese Ministry of Health and Welfare being "exclusively" manufactured as such.

Enagic International's water ionizers are also individually recognized and endorsed by the *Japanese Association of Preventive Medicine for Adult Diseases*, a renowned medical association, and are also recommended by the *Japanese Association for the Prevention of Geriatric Diseases*. The recognition and awards extend even further. Enagic has received an IEEU Environment Award from International Earth Environment University.

Enagic International is *helping people throughout the world make revolutionary, daily improvements in their lives and helping the environment*. Enagic knows how **precious** water is for human life and the magnitude of "greatness" it inherently holds.

Bless your body today with this "gift." Water your cells with Kangen® water and watch vibrant health grow. Create divine wellness within.

KANGEN® WATER REACHES:

- BLOOD STREAM in 30 seconds
- BRAIN in 1 minute
- SKIN in 10 minutes
- INTERNAL ORGANS 10 minutes

Made in the USA
Las Vegas, NV
13 June 2021